Practical taxonomic computing

Practical taxonomic computing

RICHARD J PANKHURST

Natural History Museum, London

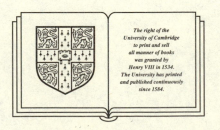

The right of the University of Cambridge to print and sell all manner of books was granted by Henry VIII in 1534. The University has printed and published continuously since 1584.

CAMBRIDGE UNIVERSITY PRESS

Cambridge

New York   Port Chester

Melbourne   Sydney

Published by the Press Syndicate of the University of Cambridge
The Pitt Building, Trumpington Street, Cambridge CB2 1RP
40 West 20th Street, New York, NY 10011-4211, USA
10 Stamford Road, Oakleigh, Victoria 3166, Australia

First published 1991

Printed in Great Britain at the University Press, Cambridge

British Library Cataloguing in Publication Data

Pankhurst, R. J. (Richard John) *1940–*
Practical taxonomic computing.
1. Taxonomy. Applications of computer systems
1. Title
574.012

ISBN 0 521 41760 0 hardback

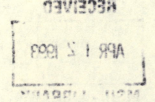

'What's the use of their having names,' the Gnat said, 'if they won't answer to them?'

'No use to *them*,' said Alice; 'but it's useful to the people that name them, I suppose. If not, why do things have names at all?'

Through the Looking Glass
Lewis Carroll

For Anne, Lucie and Thomas

Contents

Preface

The present book supersedes an earlier one. *Biological Identification* (Pankhurst, 1978) has become rapidly out of date in respect of computing techniques. The intervening ten years have seen remarkable growth in the power and availability of microcomputers. Whereas when the first book was written, only a privileged minority of biologists had the use of a computer, most of the potential users of classification and identification methods and databases will now have ready access to one. The speed and memory capacity of modern 16- or 32-bit microcomputers is now sufficient to run many of these applications on a desktop, whereas the older 8-bit machines were too small. The quality and scope of software has also greatly improved, especially for databases and graphics, which is why the book has been expanded to include these topics. More recently, the claims of expert systems have been much publicised, but it is not yet clear whether these have much to offer which has not already been anticipated by existing taxonomic software.

I acknowledge constructive criticism on the text of the new book from numerous friends and colleagues. Bob Allkin, Royal Botanic Gardens, Kew, made useful comments on the database chapter. I owe a great deal of what I have learnt about expert systems to Alex Gammerman, Department of Computer Science, Heriot-Watt University, Edinburgh. The section of cladistic classification has undergone more criticism and change than any other, as the subject is particularly controversial. My thanks here are due to Chris Hill, Department of Palaeontology; Steve Blackmore, Keeper of Botany, and Bill Sands, Department of Entomology, all at the Natural History Museum.

I have used several illustrations that appeared in *Biological Identification* and my acknowledgements are listed in the preface for that title. I would also like to thank the following for allowing the reproduction of their material:

Fig. 2.8 The Biological Records Centre.

Fig. 2.9 Flemming Skov, and the New York Botanical Garden.

R. J. Pankhurst
Natural History Museum, London
1991

Preface from
Biological Identification

This book is intended for all university students of biology, and for professional biologists who need to have some working knowledge of identification methods. It is probably the first book of its kind on this subject, as the identification of specimens is usually treated as a small section of larger textbooks on taxonomy, in spite of its considerable practical importance. There can hardly be any biologist who follows his or her career without at some stage needing to know the identity of some specimens of animals or plants which are being studied. There must be many whose daily business involves identifying specimens, but whose knowledge of taxonomy is only a means, and not an end in itself. Hence this book puts much emphasis on the practical aspects of identification methods.

An account is given of both the traditional and modern methods, and in the latter the use of a computer is often necessary. The one method with which most readers are likely to be familiar is the diagnostic key, and this is discussed in detail. On the other hand, one's view of the subject would be distorted without a proper understanding of all the other methods which have been developed in recent years. Many of these advances were only possible with the use of computers. However, those who are nervous of becoming involved with the computer ought to realise that many of the methods only require computation at a preparatory stage, and not for daily use. A short history of the subject is presented, and a brief chapter on some selected applications is provided. There is relatively little mathematics, and what there is is quite straightforward. Statistical methods are treated briefly, since practical difficulties outweigh their theoretical advantages. This is not the place to go into the details of the use of computer programs, or into the principles of computer science, and such matters are only explained in general terms. While I, personally, confess to being a botanist, I have gone to a good deal of trouble to give a balanced account suitable for biologists of all persuasions.

This book complements the following titles which have already been published by Edward Arnold*, namely *Plant Taxonomy and Biosystematics* (2nd edn), by C. Stace, and *Biological Nomenclature* (3rd edn), by Charles Jeffrey.

I wish to thank my family for their patience during the days when I shut myself away at home in order to write. I have a long-standing debt to Max Walters, Director of the Botanic Garden at Cambridge, for encouraging me to start research on

---

* Now available from Cambridge University Press.

identification methods in the first place, back in 1968, and for helping me ever since. My colleagues in the various departments of the British Museum (Natural History) have helped by numerous discussions over the past two years, and I particularly want to thank John Cannon, Keeper of Botany, for prompting me to start writing this book and for criticising the text, and Paul Whalley, Department of Entomology, for reading and criticising it too. Paul Cannon, University of Reading, and Bob Allkin, Royal Botanic Gardens, Kew, also made useful comments on the manuscript. Individual acknowledgements for permission to reproduce certain of the figures are as follows:

Fig. 4.1 Michael Chinery, and Collins Ltd.

Fig. 4.4 Paul Whalley, and the Copeland-Chatterson Co.

Fig. 4.5 Drs Hansen and Rahn, Botanical Museum, Copenhagen.

Fig. 4.6 Charles Sinker, and the Shropshire Wildlife Trust.

Fig. 4.7 Dr Nash, Western Hospital, London.

Fig. 5.5 Paul Whalley, and the British Museum (Natural History), London.

Fig. 5.6 Prof. Gyllenberg, of the Academy of Finland, the Systematics Association, and Academic Press.

Fig. 5.7 S. P. Lapage and W. R. Wilcox, and the Society for General Microbiology.

Fig. 6.1 and 6.2 The British Museum (Natural History), London.

R. J. Pankhurst
British Museum (Natural History)
1978

1

General introduction

1.1 Background

The identification of objects is a fundamental human activity. We practise it, for example, when we read the printed word, or recognise someone we know. For a biologist, identification usually means finding the name for a specimen of animal or plant, and the specimen to be identified is usually assigned to a species. Whatever sort of object is in question, it cannot be identified unless there is already a classification of like objects with which the new object can be compared. Classification here, means a way of grouping objects, on the basis of some relationship between them. The groups so formed are very often given names, and when a new object is examined, and it is decided that it belongs to one of the existing groups, then it has been identified. The purpose of these remarks is to make clear that the word 'classification' is being used in a special sense. In ordinary English, 'classify' can mean both its special sense as just given, and also it can mean 'to identify'. The verb 'to recognise' has these two meanings also. Biologists also often speak of the 'determination' of specimens, which means the same as identification, and of the 'naming' of specimens, which means identification too, but sometimes implies that this has been done temporarily or superficially.

By far the greatest part of the information which a biologist uses when identifying specimens is based on gross morphology, that is, the features that can be observed with ease, such as shape, colour and size, when the object is held in the hand. This is not because such facts are necessarily fundamental in any sense, but simply for practical reasons of speed and convenience. There is a strong tendency to avoid more specialised techniques such as dissection or microscopy, even though they may yield valuable information. Although automatic data-collecting techniques exist, most of the information used in identification is obtained by human observation and interpretation, and this seems likely to remain the case for the time being.

The diagnostic key, or 'key' for short, is by far the most frequently used identification method, and many biologists will not need an explanation of what this is. For those not familiar with it, an explanation of its use and construction is given on p.88. The key is used in most fields of biology, and its use is several centuries old. Various modern techniques are now known, which are not yet commonly applied, but which have much to commend them. This book will review both traditional and modern methods. The word 'key' is also loosely applied to identification methods other than the diagnostic key.

1.2 Some definitions

The fundamental item of information is called a *character*. Characters can be any kind of factual information which is useful in taxonomy. For example, 'flower colour' is a character for a plant. Many other words are used for the same thing, e.g. characteristic, feature, property, attribute, symptom, sign, facet and test result. Characters can be shapes, colours, sizes, chemical tests, behavioural patterns, or any information which distinguishes organisms from one another.

Characters when observed are seen to show various *states* (also called *values* or *attributes*). For example, the states of 'flower colour' might be 'red', 'white', and 'blue'. The term 'attribute' has been used variously for both 'character' and state 'state', so its use is not recommended. A character may be *constant*, if the object(s) in question have the same one and only state in all cases. If several states of a character are observed on one kind of organism, the character is *variable*. Notice that what is considered constant depends on what objects are being discussed, so this is a relative concept.

Where biology is concerned, the objects to be identified will mostly be species, or genera, or other such groupings at various levels. These are in general called *taxa* (singular *taxon*).

Characters and states are frequently combined in phrases such as 'petals white', and such an expression, consisting of a character ('petal colour') with one of its states ('white') is often loosely referred to as a 'character'. It should really be called a 'character with a state'. This distinction may seem rather a fine one, but tends to cause confusion when preparing descriptions of taxa for processing by computer. It may help to remember that a character is a noun or noun phrase, and that a state is an adjective or adjectival phrase. In the context of phylogenetic studies, 'character' is sometimes given a special meaning, i.e. 'character which has phylogenetic significance' and other characters are said not to be characters. This usage is highly confusing, and is not recommended. In what follows, 'character' will always be used in the broad sense.

Fundamental to any identification scheme is a summary of the classification on which it is based. This may be a series of written descriptions of the taxa, but is conveniently expressed as a table of taxa and characters, with the states filled in (Fig. 1.1). This is often referred to as a *taxonomic data matrix*, or just a *data matrix*. The mathematical term matrix' is only borrowed, and has little theoretical significance. The matrix is in general a rectangular one, i.e. the number of rows is not the same as the number of columns. Whether the matrix is drawn up with taxa in rows or in columns is immaterial.

For a more complete glossary of technical terms used in identification, see Morse *et al.* (1975).

1.3 Types of identification method

There are two principal kinds of method, in a broad sense, and this is true of any identification problem.

(i) *Monothetic*. This means that only one character is used at a time. The familiar diagnostic key is an example of this. Characters are used, one at a time in sequence. The identification is often achieved with only a proportion of all

CHARACTERS	1 hirsutum	2 parviflorum	3 montanum	4 lanceolatum	5 roseum	6 ciliatum	7 tetragonum ssp. tetragonum	8 tetragonum ssp. lamyi	9 obscurum	10 palustre	11 anagallidifolium	12 alsinifolium	13 brunescens
1 Habit of plant	H	E, G or H	E, G or H	E H	E H	E H	E H	E H	E H	E, G or H	D G	D G	H P
2 Stem simple hairs	S	S	A	A	A	A	A	A	A	A	*	*	A
3 Habit of stem simple hairs (if present)	+	+	–	–	+	+	+	+	–	–	–	–	–
4 Stem glandular hairs	T	T	T	L	L	L	L	L	L	T	L	L	L
5 Stem lines	–	+	–	–	–	–	–	–	–	–	–	–	+
6 Stem rooting at nodes	+	+	–	–	–	–	+	+	+	+	+	–	+
7 Stem leaves all sessile (without stalks)	semi	+	–	–	–	–	–	–	–	H	–	–	H
8 Leaves amplexicaul (clasping stem)	–	–	–	–	–	–	+	C	+	–	–	–	–
9 Leaves decurrent (running down stem)	+	–	–	–	–	–	+	C	+	–	–	–	–
10 Leaf base shape	C	R	R	C	C	R	C	C	R	C	C	R	R
11 Leaves shiny	–	–	–	–	–	–	+	+	C	C	C	+	–
12 Flower position	Te	Te	Te	Te	Te	Te	Te	Te	Te	Te	Te	Te	Ax
13 Flower diameter (mm)	15–23	6–9	6–9	6–7	4–5.5	4–5.5	6–8	10–12	7–9	4–5.5	4–5	8–9	3–4
14 Flower colour	Ro	Pi	Pi	Pi	Wp	Pi	Pi	Pi	Ro	Te	Ro	Pi	Pi
15 Stigma lobed	+	+	+	+	+	–	+	+	+	–	–	–	–
16 Stigma length relative to style	≈	∨	∨	∨	∨	∨	≈	≈	≈	∨	∨	∨	≈
17 Glandular hairs on 'calyx tube'	+	+	+	+	+	+	–	–	+	–	–	–	–
18 Fruit stalk length (cm)	0.5–1.5	0.5–1.9	0.5–1.5	1–1.9	0.5–1.9	0.5–1	0.5–1.5	0.5–1.5	0.5–1.9	1–1.9	2.5–5	2–3–5	2.5–6

Abbreviations:

A	appressed, lying against stem	H	hairy
Ax	axillary (in leaf axils, where leaves and stem join)	L	with raised lines
		P	prostrate
C	cuneate (wedge-shaped)	Pi	pink
D	decumbent to ascending i.e. stem follows ground at first, or rises at an angle	R	rounded
		Ro	rose
E	more or less erect, i.e. upright	S	spreading, standing out from stem
G	(sub)glabrous (more or less without hairs)	T	more or less terete i.e. round, without lines

Te	terminal
Wp	white to pale pink
∨	shorter, less than
≈	about equal
∧	longer, greater than
*	inapplicable
+	yes
–	no

Fig. 1.1   A data matrix for British species of *Epilobium*.

the characters which are available on the specimen. The specimen should fit exactly to the description of the taxon with which it is identified. Such identification methods may be *single access (with only one sequence and choice of characters which can be used for each specimen) or multi-access* (with any choice or sequence of characters).

(ii) *Polythetic*. This means that the method uses several characters simultaneously. An example is the tabular key (p. 105). Usually the specimen is described fairly completely before attempting identification, but it is not essential that every character of the specimen should agree with the taxon with which it is being identified.

This distinction between monothetic and polythetic methods is not hard and fast, as there are intermediate techniques (p. 109).

1.4 Hierarchies, trees and keys

Most classifications which biologists find useful are hierarchical. They consist of groups of taxa at different levels, some more general than others. Each level corresponds to a taxon, e.g. a family or genus. Each taxon can belong to only one taxon on the next higher level. This is essential if taxa are going to be identified, since an identification gives a name for labelling and reference purposes, and this is not very useful if it is ambiguous. A hierarchy can be drawn in the form of what mathematicians call a *tree*. This tree is usually drawn with its root at the top and its branches at the bottom! Fig. 1.2. illustrates a hierarchy (a classification) drawn as a tree. In this tree boxes represent taxa, and the lines show the hierarchical relationships between them, e.g. each species is connected by a line to the genus to which it belongs. By contrast, an example of a non-hierarchical classification can be given, namely that of fruit and vegetable, as in everyday use. The banana is either a fruit or a vegetable, depending on how it is used, so here is a 'taxon' which belongs to two higher groups at once, namely 'fruit' and 'vegetable'.

It is important to realise that any hierarchy can be drawn as a tree. One example already given is a classification, where we have deliberately not said anything about what sort of a classification is being represented, since there are various possibilities. One popular form of classification is that based on ancestry by evolution, known as a *phylogenetic* classification and in this case the tree representing the ancestry (called a *cladogram*) is equivalent to the classification. On the other hand, many classifications are based on observations of characters of specimens alone, and hence on their overall present-day resemblance. Such classifications are said to be *phenetic*. A tree diagram of a phenetic classification does not, therefore, necessarily correspond to an ancestry, although it may do so. It is sometimes called a *dendrogram*. There has been much controversy over whether the phylogenetic or phenetic approach is the proper one to use, but this will not be discussed here. For further reading, contrast the views of Sneath and Sokal (1974) with those of Hennig (1966).

Lastly, the popular identification key, or diagnostic key, can also be drawn as a tree, where the boxes represent the decisions to be taken, and only the boxes on the final branches represent taxa. Fig. 1.3 represents the same key as in Figs 1.4 and 1.5, but expressed as a tree. Hence the tree of a key is something different again. Some authors like to construct keys which reflect

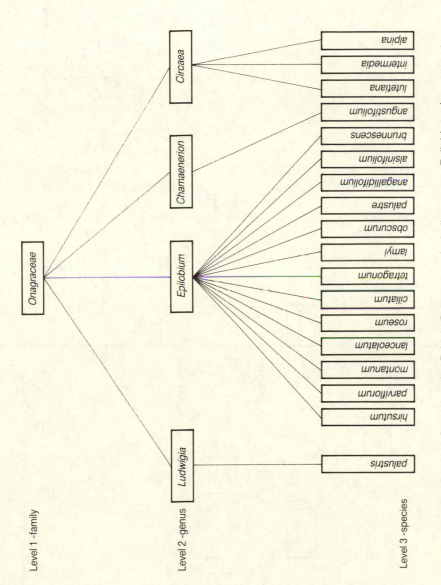

Fig. 1.2 Classification of some native British *Onagraceae*, including genus *Epilobium*, drawn as a tree.

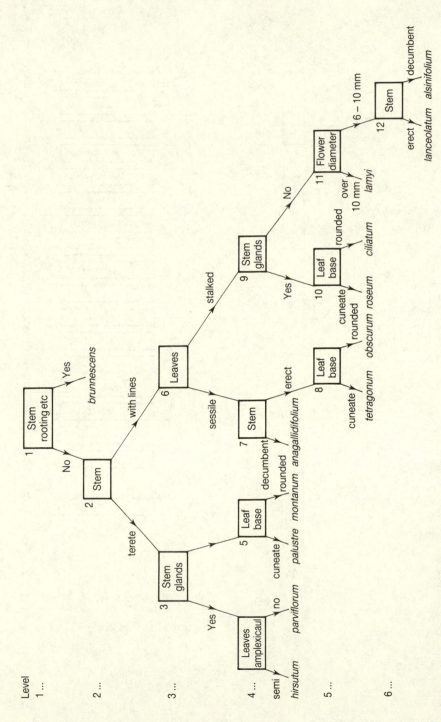

Fig. 1.3   Simplified *Epilobium* key drawn as a tree.

1	Stem rooting at nodes, prostrate, flowers axillary.	*brunnescens*
	Stem not rooting at nodes, decumbent, ascending or erect, flowers terminal	2
2(1)	Stem more or less terete	3
	Stem with raised lines	6
3(2)	Stem with glandular hairs	4
	Stem without glandular hairs	5
4(3)	Leaves semi-amplexicaul and decurrent, cuneate at base, flowers over 10 mm diam., petals rose	*hirsutum*
	Leaves not amplexicaul, nor decurrent, rounded at base, flowers 6–10 mm diam., petals pink	*parviflorum*
5(3)	Leaf cuneate at base, flowers under 6 mm diam., stigma entire	*palustre*
	Leaf rounded at base, flowers 6–10 mm diam., stigma 4-lobed	*montanum*
6(2)	Leaves more or less sessile	7
	At least some leaves stalked	9
7(6)	Stem decumbent to ascending, subglabrous, flowers under 6 mm diam., fruit stalk 2–5 cm	*anagallidifolium*
	Stem more or less erect, with simple hairs, flowers 6–10 mm diam., fruit stalk under 2 cm	8
8(7)	Leaf cuneate at base, shiny above, glandular hairs absent from 'calyx tube', petals pink	*tetragonum*
	Leaf rounded at base, dull above, glandular hairs present on 'calyx tube', petals rose	*obscurum*
9(6)	Stem with glandular hairs, flowers under 6 mm diam.	10
	Stem without glandular hairs, flowers over 6 mm diam.	11
10(9)	Leaf cuneate at base, petals white to pale pink, stigma more or less equal to style	*roseum*
	Leaf rounded at base, petals pink, stigma less than style	*ciliatum*
11(9)	Flowers over 10 mm diam.	*lamyi*
	Flowers 6–10 mm diam.	12
12(11)	Stem more or less erect, with simple hairs, leaf cuneate at base, stigma 4-lobed, fruit stalk under 2 cm	*lanceolatum*
	Stem decumbent to ascending, subglabrous, leaf rounded at base, stigma entire, fruit stalk 2–5 cm	*alsinifolium*

Fig. 1.4 Key to British *Epilobium* species, parallel style.

1	Stem rooting at nodes, prostrate, flowers axillary.	*brunnescens*
1*	Stem not rooting at nodes, decumbent, ascending or erect, flowers terminal	2
2	Stem more or less terete	3
3	Stem with glandular hairs	4
4	Leaves semi-amplexicaul and decurrent, cuneate at base, flowers over 10 mm diam., petals rose	*hirsutum*
4*	Leaves not amplexicaul, not decurrent, rounded at base, flowers 6–10 mm diam., petals pink	*parviflorum*
3*	Stem without glandular hairs	5
5	Leaf cuneate at base, flowers under 6 mm diam., stigma entire	*palustre*
5*	Leaf rounded at base, flowers 6–10 mm diam., stigma 4-lobed	*montanum*
2*	Stem with raised lines	6
6	Leaves more or less sessile	7
7	Stem decumbent to ascending, subglabrous, flowers under 6 mm diam. fruit stalk 2–5 cm	*angallidifolium*
7*	Stem more or less erect with simple hairs, flowers 6–10 mm diam., fruit stalk under 2 cm	8
8	Leaf cuneate at base, shiny above, glandular hairs absent from 'calyx tube', petals pink	*tetragonum*
8*	Leaf rounded at base, dull above, glandular hairs present on 'calyx tube', petals rose	*obscurum*
6*	At least some leaves stalked	9
9	Stem with glandular hairs, flowers under 6 mm diam.	10
10	Leaf cuneate at base, petals white to pale pink, stigma more or less equal to style	*roseum*
10*	Leaf rounded at base, petals pink, stigma less than style	*ciliatum*
9*	Stem without glandular hairs, flowers over 6 mm diam.	11
11	Flowers over 10 mm diam.	*lamyi*
11*	Flowers 6–10 mm diam.	12
12	Stem more or less erect, with simple hairs, leaf cuneate at base, stigma 4-lobed, fruit stalk under 2 cm	*lanceolatum*
12*	Stem decumbent to ascending, subglabrous, leaf rounded at base, stigma entire, fruit stalk 2–5 cm	*alsinifolium*

Fig. 1.5   Key to British *Epilobium* species, yoked style.

the classification, and these are called *natural* keys. The tree of a key made this way may look very much like the dendrogram or cladogram on which it is based, as characters or combinations of characters can always be chosen from the taxa in order to do this. However, such keys tend to require the use of several characters in combination, any or all of which are often qualified by adjectives such as 'usually' and 'sometimes'. As a result, a natural key is harder to use and less reliable than the *artificial* key. An artificial key is based on whatever characters are easiest to observe and which produce the answer most quickly and reliably. It therefore need not bear any obvious resemblance to the classification to which it corresponds.

The natural key is a way of setting out a classification and it is not recommended simply for the practical purpose of obtaining fast, reliable identification. From this point onward, by 'key' we shall understand 'artificial key'. It is evident that when one wishes to identify a specimen, one must proceed with the characters it presents on the basis that no knowledge is available, at that moment, of the phylogenetic relationships of the species to which it belongs. In this sense, all identifications are necessarily phenetic. It is possible for a species to evolve in such a way that it has a close but superficial resemblance to another species to which it is not very closely related by ancestry. This is known as *convergent evolution*. A phylogenetic classification involving two such species should separate them to a degree which reflects their origin, and not their present-day similarity. On the other hand, an efficient key for identifying these two species must deal with them together, since they are rather alike. It is also possible that the characters which are thought to be significant for phylogeny and which are presented in a classification are not the same as those which are convenient for identification. These remarks show how principles of classification can conflict with the practical needs of identification. For the purposes of the remainder of this book, the classification of a group of organisms will be taken for granted, without regard to methods by which it is created, as a starting point for identification problems.

1.5 Pattern recognition

Pattern recognition is a general term for the application of computers to problems of recognition. The relation of this subject to the identification of biological specimens is briefly discussed in this section.

Pattern recognition methods are applied to a great diversity of problems, including biological applications. As a broad generalisation, one can say that much pattern recognition work has an extra complement which is missing from the conventional practice of identification by biologists, because the object to be recognised is very frequently *digitised* at a preliminary stage. This means that electronic equipment (such as a video camera, or a pencil follower) is first used to obtain a representation of the object of interest. This representation is sometimes a table of values of lightness or darkness over an area, or a sequence of geometrical co-ordinates for positions on a line. In other words, the description of the object to be identified is obtained automatically in a form that a computer can handle by automatic processes. This is very much in contrast with a biologist identifying a specimen, who will mostly make his or her own observations, and then draw conclusions, without much direct use of any equipment (except perhaps a microscope).

Once the description of an object has been stored in a computer, the stage of *feature extraction* still has to take place. This is the equivalent of recognising the shape of a leaf of a plant, or counting the number of antennal segments on an insect. What a human observer perceives in a few seconds can be a complex process for a computer to perform. A further difficulty is the physical complexity of natural organisms, with the variations of growth in any one species, and in the problems of dealing with a three-dimensional object seen from an arbitrary direction. The more successful uses of computers in pattern recognition often concern objects which are relatively simple, e.g. only objects with regular edges and surfaces in the analysis of pictures, or those which have only two dimensions, such as the karyology of human chromosomes, or recognition of handwriting. For a general introduction to pattern recognition see Mendel and Fu (1970). For the time being, it seems likely that most identifications of plants and animals will depend on human observation (but see Chapter 3, p. 159).

This is not the place to go into the theory of pattern recognition, but some useful comments can be made. For any polythetic identification method which calculates a measure of similarity by adding to the measure for each character which agrees, it is possible to use a numerical weighting for each character in the hope of improving the results (see p. 142). There is a theorem which shows that if such a method is used, and if there exists a set of weights which will give the correct identification with a set of samples, then it is always possible to compute those weights. This result is known as the *perceptron convergence theorem* (Minsky and Papert, 1969). Put in other words, if correct identification by such a method is possible, then the necessary character weights can always be calculated. One can find a set of examples and calculate the weights and then use the weights to identify more samples, calculate the weights again, and so on. The significance of this is that it is a learning process, and if carried out by computer, what is taking place is a process of *artificial intelligence*, since a computer program has altered its behaviour as a result of experience. This is one of the important aspects of human intelligence.

2

Databases

2.1 Introduction

A *database* may be defined as data which has *structure* together with some *system* for organising it. The system in question is usually a computer. If data possess structure this alone is not enough to make a database. Consider an index of addresses consisting of a drawer full of cards. Each card has a person's name on the top line, say, with the postal address written below. This data does therefore have some formal structure, but it has no general system for retrieving information and is not a database in the above sense. The only kind of query which can be easily answered with this system is to find the address given the name. If the problem was to find a person's name given their address, the only way to do it would be to search every card by hand. On the other hand, a personal letter prepared with a word processor will not have a great deal of structure, apart from sentences and paragraphs, but the word processing program provides a complex system for handling it, so that it is a system without structure, and again not a database. For the sake of complete accuracy it is necessary to say that so-called unstructured database systems do exist, but that in such cases the structure is added or imposed internally at a later stage, so that structure is still necessary, even if it is not immediately visible.

2.2 Databases for taxonomy

What do databases have to do with biological taxonomy? The main products of taxonomic research are published floras, faunas and monographs. A *flora* is a book containing des-criptions of the plants which grow in a given geographical area, together with identification keys for naming them, and summaries of other relevant facts, such as distribution and ecology. A *fauna* is an equivalent publication for animals. A *monograph* deals with a particular group of animals or plants, sometimes for a limited geographical area, and provides similar information, although often in greater detail. Such publications usually contain the following data:

1) a list of the taxa present in the area, with their various names;
2) a description of each taxon, more or less sufficient to distinguish each one from the rest;
3) brief summaries of other data, such as habitat, distribution and ecology;
4) some means of identifying specimens, usually diagnostic keys.

These kinds of publications have highly structured data, but usually lack any system, in the sense given above. As a result, although relevant information may be present, it often cannot be easily extracted. Examples of this are:

1) analysis of data of almost any kind between unrestricted selections of different groups of taxa. In particular, it is very difficult to compare any properties of the taxa unless they are closely related. It is usually not practicable to make maps of any taxonomic data over some geographical region. Similarly, it is often not practicable to select taxa which share some special property, e.g. medicinal plants;

2) the use of alternative classifications of the taxa other than the classification which is provided;

3) the identification of specimens is restricted to mature and complete examples. For example, identification of vegetative plant specimens is usually impossible.

In the following discussion, it should become apparent that as and when taxonomic data are converted into databases, it becomes much more accessible and useful. Various textbooks describe how taxonomic data is collected and processed, but the clearest account available, for plants at any rate, is by Leenhouts (1968). The details of what data is required and how exactly it will be processed depend on the particular project, but several broad categories of information may be recognised (Pankhurst, 1988a), as follows.

1) Curatorial data, essentially the information given on labels of preserved specimens, such as the scientific name(s) given to the specimen, geographical data stating where the specimen was collected, when and by whom, plus any notes on habitat and morphology.

2) Distribution data for taxa, in terms of geographical coordinates or political or other areas in which taxa occur.

3) Nomenclatural data, comprising the scientific name(s), details of the publication and the author(s), and references to type specimen(s), if known. It may be important to distinguish between taxa whose names are considered valid (accepted names), and other names, such as synonyms.

4) Bibliographical data, including the names, authors and dates of relevant publications in books and journals, with possibly some indication of the nature of the information.

5) Morphological data. In the wider sense this may include not merely descriptions of the physical appearance of organisms but also other types of data such as chemistry and cytology.

Taxonomic data may be classified in other ways. In particular, it may be useful to consider whether the data is oriented towards specimens (curatorial) or taxa (most of the rest). A further distinction can be made between data which is explicitly based on valid taxa (accepted names) or on other names as well. The categories of taxonomic data have a tendency to overlap and interlink. In particular, much of the data about taxa ultimately depends on data from specimens, e.g. geographical distribution, and morphology.

Taxonomic data are collected, sorted and sifted and then processed to produce taxonomic publications, usually in book form. The whole process has been described as an information service (Bisby, 1984). The book format imposes a number of very important limitations.

1) Information can only be searched for via the index given the names of taxa. There is no effective means to search for data based on other criteria.

2) Much useful data is absent simply because it is too expensive to publish it. Worse, the information presented may be just an author's opinion based on data which is not available for inspection or further use. The lack of publication or preservation of voluminous but important data often leads to work being wastefully repeated at a later date.

3) Pictorial information such as illustrations and maps is not generally published, because of expense, and this is all the more true when colour is involved. Nevertheless, there are vast stores of original images such as drawings, paintings and photographs in collections and libraries which are scarcely used except by staff or visitors to the institutes which own them, because of the difficulty of making them generally available. To these must be added images of specimens or parts of specimens.

Both the source data and the published products comprise structured data, and require only to be placed into a computer database system in order to become full and proper databases, with all the attendant advantages. Via the use of external computer memory (e.g. magnetic or optical discs) there is now the possibility of preserving and disseminating all the useful taxonomic data at modest expense.

2.3 Definitions

The important features of a computerised database system which is to handle the data are as follows:

1) *Random access*, which means that it should be more or less equally easy to reach all parts of the data, and in any order.

2) *Multiple indexing*. An *index* is simply a list of data items together with a pointer to where the data is to be found. In the familiar example of an index in a book, the pointers are page numbers. The card index of addresses referred to above is self-indexing, if the cards are kept in alphabetical order of the names. Museum collections of animals or plants are often kept in systematic order, according to families and genera, and such collections are also self-indexed. Within such a collection there might then be a secondary ordering according to geographical areas. If you are looking for a plant from a particular country and you know its name, then there is no problem. If, on the other hand, you wanted to find all specimens collected by a certain person before a certain date, then the question would be very tedious or impractical to answer. With a computerised database acting as a catalogue to a collection, there would be no more difficulty in answering the second of these questions than the first, provided that suitable indexes had been set up.

3) *Sorting* database information in alphabetical, numerical or date order is a very simple process by computer. It is also easy to sort on more than one criterion, just by repeating the process. For example, to get a list of species in order alphabetically by genus and species, the computer will sort first by species and then by genus. Notice that the actual order in which this is done is reversed, although the database system will often accept the sorting instructions in the intuitive order.

4) *Retrieval* of information and the preparation of *reports* from a computer database is generally very rapid. This means that it is relatively easy to extract data for special purposes, and to make reports or publications from selected information. Searching for information in a database, or *information retrieval*,

may mean no more than looking for all occurrences of a certain name or other string of symbols by direct searching and comparison, such as most word-processing programs are capable of doing. However, the structuring of data means that the location for certain kinds of information is known in advance and it is this that can make the retrieval of information from a well organised database so very effective. Often the data which is contained in a database changes with time, and the usefulness of the database depends on keeping it up to date. The maintenance of a database will require the correction or *editing* of existing data and *updating* by the addition of new data. If such updating is regularly carried out, then there is the great advantage that up-to-date information is always available.

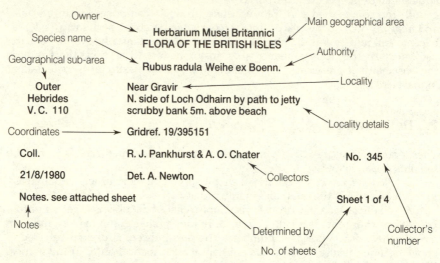

Fig. 2.1 A typical herbarium specimen label.

A database *record* or *row* is a repeating group of data items. For example, an entry in a telephone directory might be a record. The items within each entry include the name, address and telephone number. The information on specimen labels in a natural history collection could also be a record. A record is sometimes also known as a *tuple*, but this strictly only applies to a relational database (see below). There can sometimes be confusion over the meaning of the word 'record', especially in the context of biological recording, where to say that there is 'record' for an organism means that note has been taken of its occurrence in a particular locality. If this information is stored in a database, then there is a record (biological sense) which is being kept in a record (database sense). When there is more than one record these may be kept in a *table* with a number of rows or entries, and each record could be identified by its sequential position or *record number*. A *field* or *column* is a subdivision of a record, containing data of one kind only. In the specimen label (Fig. 2.1) there is, amongst others, a field for the name(s) of the collector(s) and another for the date of collection. Fields are sometimes given a *type*, as one means to permit checking of correct data entry. As an example, the collector's name might be of type 'alphabetic string' and the date could be of type 'date'. A field might be of fixed or variable length. The collector's name field would naturally vary in length, as some names are longer than others, but it might be necessary to decide in advance how long the longest name could be, in order to reserve sufficient computer memory for it. The date field could have a fixed length, provided that day, month and year were always known, and it could also have a fixed *format*, such as for example, two digits (day) followed by period followed by three letters (month), another period and four digits (year). Fields might repeat and have subfields, such as for example the collector might be two or more persons, and there might be a subfield for each name. The field is then said to be *multivalued*. In a database system which does not allow multivalued fields, data of this kind would be expressed as multiple rows in an additional table. It is possible for fields to be *coded*, i.e. to substitute a number or letter code for the data in the field. For example, a reference list of numbers for known names of collectors might be used and the number stored in the place of the name. The list of names and numbers might also be stored in a separate part of the database. A list of this kind may be presented as a menu, when it is called a *choice list*. It is usually necessary to be able to identify each record uniquely, and a *key* field may be defined for this purpose. The word 'key' here has a different meaning from 'key' in the sense of an identification key. In the example of a collection label, it may be that every specimen has a unique accession number, and this could be used as a key field. Failing this, it may be necessary to invent a key field for each record, or alternatively, a record key may be defined as some unique combination of the contents of two or more other fields. With botanical collections, it is often possible to identify each specimen uniquely by a combination of collector's name and collector's number. The term *data dictionary* is sometimes used to describe collectively the names and other properties of all the fields in a record and to refer to where this information is stored.

An *index* has the same function in a database as it has in a book. A book might have a contents list at the front, where the subjects are listed in order of the page numbers. The page number is here the key, in the database sense, which uniquely identifies each page. The index at the back of the book has an alphabetical list of subjects with the corresponding page number(s), and may well contain much of the same information as the contents list does. The difference is mainly in the ordering of the information. The contents list is ordered numerically by page and the index is ordered alphabetically by subject. The original ordering by key field (page number) has been inverted. In a computer, an index will list the keys for the records according to the contents of a field or fields which are indexed. In a computerised database there can be as many indices as are needed, and several can be used together so that any combination of information can be retrieved quickly. Indices are often used for sorting, since it is more practical to create or copy an index to the data of interest and to sort that, than to sort the actual records.

Database systems, whether relational or not, will normally provide some means of controlling access to the database and providing security. The database may be partitioned in areas that certain users may see and alter and others not, or the type of access may be controlled, e.g. read only. Users may have to give a password before being allowed to use the database. These considerations may not be of much importance in databases used for scientific research, where the data is often neither private nor sensitive.

2.4 Data structures

A *data structure* is the organisation of data in a computer memory. The simplest data item is a single constant or *variable* which is identified inside the computer by a single address. An example might be a variable for the 'height of a stem'. A slightly more complicated structure is the *array*, which is a number of variables, all of the same kind, distinguished by a subscript or index. An example might be the stem heights for 20 different plants, numbered 1 to 20. The same idea can be generalised to arrays with two or more subscripts. An array with two subscripts is the equivalent of a table (matrix), with data values in the rows and columns, all of the same kind. If the data referred to 20 different properties of the stem for one plant, instead of the same property for 20 different plants, then the structure is really just the same as that of a database record, as defined above. The same kind of data structure occurs in the C programming language (Kernigan and Ritchie, 1978) where it is simply called a 'structure'.

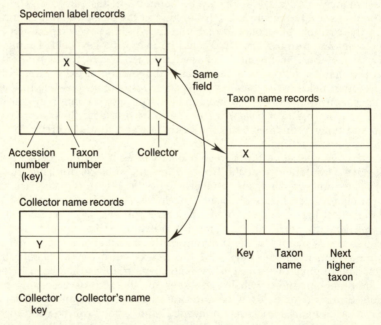

Fig. 2.2   Blocks in a relational data structure.

So far the data structures which have been described only contain data, and are complete in themselves. Each of the above data structure units could be used as a *block* which forms part of a larger structure. In order to arrange this, some data fields must contain not raw data, but a reference to other blocks. This reference could be some kind of *pointer*, i.e. the address of another part of memory, or the number of a record in another block. In particular, the contents of the key field of a record could be used to refer to that record from elsewhere, since that is unique. It is not a good idea to use the record number for this purpose, since the order in which the records are kept might very well change. An example of this kind of data structure is shown in Fig. 2.2. The records in the main table are from specimen labels such as that in Fig 2.1. The first field (column) is to be the accession number of the specimen, which is unique and can therefore serve as a key. The next field will represent the species name. This field could of course simply contain that name, spelt out in full, but instead a number X is inserted to represent that species. X is the same as the contents of a key field in a record in a separate table for species names, and the reference is indicated by an arrow. The full name of the species is spelt out in the second table. In a similar way, the name of the person who collected the specimen is represented by the reference number Y in another field in the main table which refers to a record in a third table for names of collectors. This kind of data structure might be described as a set of linked tables. There is an infinite number of ways in which data structures can be constructed. Another possible arrangement would be a hierarchy of linked tables. This might be used to represent a taxonomic hierarchy of nomenclature, where the top table is for families, the next for genera, and a third for species. Such a data structure has the same general appearance as the *tree* illustrated in Fig. 1.2, although the details are not the same. Yet another possibility is to have a number of blocks which are connected in a network, so that any block is or could be connected to any other. According to current thinking, all these various kinds of data structure are most efficiently represented for database processing by one particular general structure, which is known as a *relational database*. The structure in Fig. 2.2, as discussed above, is a particular example of it.

2.5 Relational databases

A formal definition of a relational database exists (e.g. Codd, 1970; Date, 1981) but it will not be helpful to explore this in detail. Many commercially available database systems, which are claimed to be relational, fall far short of the proper definition, and may provide nothing more than the means to manipulate linked tables. The important features of a relational database system are as follows.

1) The means to process data in linked tables. To say that the tables are linked means that fields of one table refer to data in records of other tables, as in the example just discussed. To process the data means that it must be possible to create and alter the definitions of the tables and their contents.

2) Each item of data is stored only once, and only referred to in one way, even though it may be referred to many times. This simple rule, which can apply equally well to any kind of database, will ensure that when changes and corrections are made, there will be no problem of having to find and alter data in many different places. Any update will only have to be made once. Another implication of this is that no table may contain the same record more than once. An important consequence of the rule about each data item only appearing once is economy of memory usage. In the specimen label example of Fig. 2.2, the scientific name of the organism was represented by a reference to another table. It could have been simply entered in a field or fields of the main table, so why not do that? The reason is that the name can occur more than once. There could be hundreds of specimens in the collection which

have that same name. The number X which replaces the name and gives its record number in another table is likely to be far shorter than the name spelt out in full, and so there is considerable space saving. Also, when the name changes, as they so often do, only one entry in the species name table needs to be altered.

3) Data independence. The idea is that it should not matter which medium the data is stored on, and that programs which relate to the database should not have to be altered when the data changes. This is again a property to be desired in any database system, whether relational or not. It is certainly possible to achieve this when it is only a matter of altering data within fields, but when the definition of the tables is changed, by adding new tables and new fields, then it is more likely that the programs must change to take account of this. Whether data independence is possible or not is partly a matter of how applications of the database system are designed as well as being a property of the system itself.

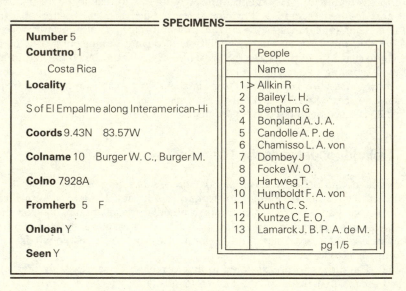

Fig. 2.3   Data capture screen for specimen data.

4) A well designed system will ensure that coding of fields, if necessary, is done internally, and not externally by somebody who has to mentally look up a number or letter code. This will avoid numerous opportunities for making mistakes. As an example, with the database of Fig. 2.2, there will be a moment during data entry when it is necessary to key in the collector(s) names(s). Ideally these should be presented as a menu on a display from which the correct name is selected with a single key, as in Fig. 2.3. If the appropriate name is not in the menu, then there should be a simple way to enter a new name and have the menu brought up to date.

2.6 An example database

The PANDORA database will be used as a concrete example with which to illustrate the uses of databases for taxonomy. The database is designed to help the writer of a flora to handle relevant data about specimens, taxa (nomenclature), publications (bibliography), geographical distribution, and morphological descriptions. An early version of this database was developed with the dBASEIII system (Pankhurst, 1988a), but has now been transferred to Advanced Revelation (COSMOS, 1987). Various examples from this database will be used to illustrate this chapter. The different files (tables) used in this database and the relations between them are shown in Fig. 2.4. There are three files which depend on no others. These are:

HERBARIUM, with a list of herbarium codes and addresses,
PERSONS, with people's names, and
CHARACTERS, with a list of descriptive characters.

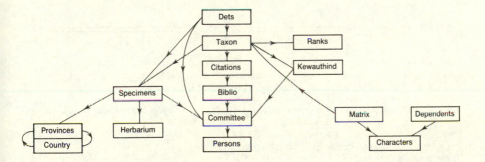

Fig. 2.4   Diagram of database file structure.

People are referred to in a number of different contexts, because their names occur as collectors of specimens, as authors of taxa, as names on determination labels which say who named a specimen as what, and as authors and editors of books and journal articles. The same people may and do appear in more than one of these contexts, so their names should only be stored once. As a further complication, people work in groups as collectors or authors, and the order in which their names appear may be significant. In order to allow for this, there is a file called COMMITTEE which records which persons have worked together and the order of their names. In order to have a uniform way to refer to all persons, whether for some project they were working on by themselves or with others, a COMMITTEE record can refer to just one person. Although any reference to people's names will in fact be stored in COMMITTEE and linked from there to PERSONS, all this mechanism is hidden from users of the database, who will only see the actual person's name.

The file COUNTRY keeps a list of all country names, and points to PROVINCES for a list of the provinces (states, counties etc.) for each. The table PROVINCES keeps a list of provinces for each country. The SPECIMENS file contains one record for each herbarium specimen, which may be an actual

```
═══════════════════════ TAXON ═══════════════════════
│                                                              │
│  Number . .                        Name. type  . . . . .      │
│                                                              │
│  Taxon. name  . . . . . . . . . . . . . . . . . .   Rank. no.  . . . . . . .  │
│                                                              │
│  Next. higher. taxon  . . . . . . . . . . . . . .             │
│                                                              │
│  Authority  . . . . . . . . . . . . . . . . . . . . .         │
│                                                              │
│  Family  . . . . . . . . . . . . . . . . . . . . .           │
│                                                              │
│  Genus  . . . . . . . . . . . . . . . . . . . . . .          │
│                                                              │
│  Species  . . . . . . . . . . . . . . . . . . . . .          │
│                                                              │
│  Type. sp. no.  . . . . . . . . . . . . . . . . .   Type. type  . . . . . .   │
│                                                              │
│  Type. cit . . . . . . . . . . . . . . . . . . . . .         │
│                                                              │
│  Synonym. type  . . . . . . . . . . . . . . . .   Synonym. of . . . . .      │
│                                                              │
│  Synonym. list . . . . . . . . . . . . . . . . . . .         │
│                                                              │
══ Default value is 69 ═══════════════════════════════
```

Number   Record key   **Name. type**   Accepted, synonym etc.
Taxon. name   The name e.g. 'annua', 'Rosaceae' at some level
Rank. no.   The level of the taxon. name e.g. species, family, variety
Authority   Author(s) name(s) and key to authority file
Next. higher. taxon   Key to next higher taxon e.g. if Taxon. name is a species, this may
                          point to a genus
Family, Genus, Species   Names computed from Next. higher. taxon
Type. sp. no   Key in SPECIMENS file for a type specimen
Type. type   What kind of type e.g. HOLO-, SYN-
Type. cit   Literature citation to where Taxon. name published
Synonym. type   Only if Name. type = synonym e.g. partial, pro parte
Synonym. of   If Name. type = synonym, points to accepted name(s)
Synonym. list   If Name. type not synonym, list of synonymous names

Fig. 2.5   Data capture screen for nomenclature.

specimen available for examination or just the details of a specimen copied from a publication. If there are duplicate specimens (probably in different herbaria or museums) then each specimen gets a different entry, since it can be labelled differently, and may show different characters. Each specimen record refers to the COUNTRY and PROVINCES (if known), and stores the locality details, date of collection, altitude and latitude-longitude, collector name(s) and number (via COMMITTEE), the herbarium (via HERBARIUM) which owns the specimen and notes whether the specimen has been seen for the project and whether it has been borrowed or not.

The BIBLIO file keeps record of each separate bibliographic source. This refers to authors and editors of publications via COMMITTEE. Since a source such as a flora or journal may be referenced more than once, there is a separate CITATIONS file to store details such as volume and page number and this also refers to BIBLIO to give the source. It is customary to abbreviate the names of authors of taxa when the scientific names are quoted, e.g. *Poa annua* L., where the L. is an abbreviation for Carl Linnaeus. For plants, these abbreviations are more or less standardised and the reference used for these is Meikle (1980). Once again, more than one person may be involved, so the abbreviation is stored in the KEWAUTHIND file as well as the COMMITTEE number. These files are all needed as a basis for the nomenclature data in the TAXON file. This contains the name and its level, e.g. family, genus, species and lower level names (if needed) and a reference to the next higher taxon to which this name belongs (see Fig. 2.5). There is a reference to KEWAUTHIND in order to give the taxon author(s) names, and a reference to SPECIMENS in order to define the type specimen (if known) and to CITATIONS in order to state where and when the taxon was published. Finally, the DETS file records the names given to specimens. Some specimens have been labelled with different names by different people at different times, and the latest name is supposed to be the right one. However, it is not safe to assume that the latest name is necessarily correct, and it is useful to be able to trace specimens named by a particular expert. Hence DETS refers to SPECIMENS and to COMMITTEE, and can have more than one record for each specimen but with different dates or persons. The files for the descriptions all depend on the list of CHARACTERS. The MATRIX file depends on both the CHARACTERS and the TAXON files. A separate file called DEP stores the dependencies between characters.

2.7 Data capture and updating

The phrase *data capture* refers to the process of collecting data and adding it to the database. The use of the word 'capture' helps to emphasise that data collection can be both laborious and difficult. Nevertheless, good design of the database system and of the application can make data capture much easier. In some applications, it may be necessary to prepare a paper *form* or questionnaire, on which data are entered manually in a separate stage before it is entered into a computer. It is far better to avoid this, if possible, since it means that the data has to be prepared twice, once on the forms and again when entered in a computer. Also, the form filling stage allows many errors to be introduced since there is no computer controlling the validity of the data, and the extra stage of copying doubles the opportunities for making factual errors by miscopying. In some circumstances, forms may be necessary when the computer cannot be brought close to the source of data, but even so, the use of a portable computer is still a better solution. Fig. 2.6 shows an example of a form used by the Flora Veracruz project for label data.

In the past, data had to be entered in fixed positions on punched cards, but modern database systems will provide for a data entry screen on a display. This screen is also sometimes referred to as a form, by analogy with the paper version, and the layout of such a screen may be called a template. Fig. 2.5 illustrates a data capture screen for the TAXON file of nomenclatural data from the PANDORA database.

This particular screen has been set up to collect data on the scientific names of plant taxa, including the actual Latin names, the status of the name, the author(s) of the taxon, and details about the type specimen. In the following explanations, many of the details are specific to the particular database system, which happens to be a sophisticated one, so other database systems need not be expected to perform in exactly the same way. When

INSTITUTO NACIONAL DE INVESTIGACIONES SOBRE RECURSOS BIOTICOS

HERBARIO   FLORA DE MEXICO   FLORA DE VERACRUZ

No. Rec. Inf/1/_____ Clave/2/_____ Fam./3/_____

Nombre Científico/4/ _____

País/5/_____ Estado/6/_____ Mun./7/_____

Localidad/8/ _____

_____ Mapa/9/_____

Lat./10/_____ Long./11/_____ Alt/12/_____

Tip. Veg./13/_____ Prim. ( ) Sec. ( ) /14/____

Inf Ambiental/15/ _____

Suelo/16/ _____

_____

Asociada/17/ _____

Abund./18/_____ Forma Biol./19/_____ Tamaño/20/_____

An. ( ) Perenne ( ) /21/ Otros Datos/30/ _____

Fruto/22/_____ Flor/23/_____

Nom. Loc/24/_____ Fecha Col./25/_____

Usos/26/_____ Det./27/_____

Col./28/_____ No/29/_____

Her./31/_____ Dupl./32/_____

Fig. 2.6 Flora Veracruz data entry form.

the screen is selected, it is assumed that the user means to enter an entirely new record. It happens in this case that the records are given numbers in sequence, and the system has been set up so that it will suggest the next unused number as a default. This appears on the bottom line with the statement "Default value is 69". The flashing cursor will be initially positioned over the dotted line after the first field (Number), waiting for the user to type a new record number. In order to accept the default which is offered, it is only necessary to hit the Enter key and the number 69 will go into the Number field. The cursor then automatically moves to the next field, called Name.type. This is used to record the status of the name, such as whether it is accepted, synonymous, provisional etc. A single letter is used to indicate one of these. Data validation is set up for this field, so that if the user types anything other than A or S or P (or a or s or p), an error message will appear, saying what is wrong. This is an example of how the computer can actually help during the process of data collection by preventing the entry of anything other than the right kind of data. It cannot, of course, detect the mistake if you type an A when it should have been an S, since either is legal. While either upper or lower case letters can be typed for this field, they are actually all converted and stored in upper case for the sake of internal consistency. The next field, and probably the most important one, is the Taxon.name. This is best explained by means of an example. Consider the name *'Bellis perennis'* (actually the Common Daisy). This species belongs to the family Compositae, also known as the Asteraceae, but this fact is not explicitly stated in the name. In order to enter this name completely, at least three different records are needed; one for *'Bellis'*, another for *'perennis'* and a third for 'Compositae'. The following field, called Next.higher.taxon is used to show the connection. For *'perennis'* the next higher taxon is *'Bellis'*, and similarly, *'Bellis'* is referred to 'Compositae'. The next field is called Rank.no, and this is used to indicate the level of the Taxon.name, e.g. genus, species, cultivar etc. There is a choice of about twenty different levels. It is a mistake if this field is not filled in, and if the user tries to leave it empty and skip it, the computer will refuse. This is an example of a field which is set up to be obligatory or mandatory, and so it is not possible to make the mistake of leaving it out. Since the user is likely to be entering a series of records for the same genus, this field has also been given a default, which offers the same value as in the last record entered. In other words, the user can say 'ditto' in order to repeat the same rank as before, without having to type an identical field repeatedly.

The next field, Authority, illustrates another principle. The authority for a plant name is the person or persons who originally published the taxon and this is abbreviated in a stylised way. The official authority abbreviation and the actual names of the persons involved are stored in the KEWAUTHIND, COMMITTEE and PERSONS files. This is because all of these can be and are referred to repeatedly in other tables, and so should only be entered once. The field Authority only needs to contain a reference to the KEWAUTHIND file, and its record key is used for this. How then does the user know what to put for this field? Clearly he does not want to have to separately go to a screen for author abbreviations and look up the record key from there, and should not be expected to somehow know what the key is already. Instead, the system is set up to provide a menu or *choice list*. This appears automatically as soon as the Authority field is reached, and offers a choice of the acceptable abbreviations expressed in words and in alphabetical order. Because of the way that a choice list appears or 'pops up' when it is needed, it is sometimes referred to as a *pop-up*. The correct abbreviation is chosen from the menu by using the arrow key pad, and the computer looks up the right record key. This key and the abbreviation in words are then both put on the screen for the Author field. Once again, the computer makes sure that only correct abbreviations are entered, and also saves the user from having to type them out.

A procedure has just been described so that data from one table can be referred to whilst entering data into another. What happens, however, if that data is not already there? In the above example, what if the authority that is to be entered is not already on the choice list? Obviously, a data capture screen for KEWAUTHIND, and possibly also one for PERSONS, need to be accessed, and ideally without abandoning the screen for taxa which is currently being used. At first sight, this looks like a disadvantage of the relational structure, since not all the data is accessible at one time, and there are times when it is necessary to look at more than one table at once. In some database systems it will be necessary to save the incomplete record and exit the current screen in order to go to other screens in order to fill in the missing information, before returning to the incomplete original record in order to complete it. The better systems will allow 'nesting' of screens, so that when in the middle of the taxon screen, for example, it is possible to hit a special key on the keyboard and hence call up other screens such as authority abbreviations and persons, and return to the taxon screen afterwards in the same place as before, and without any data being lost. It may even be possible to call up one screen from within another repeatedly, i.e. to have multiple levels of nesting.

Returning to the screen in Fig. 2.5, the next field is for Type.sp.no, i.e. type specimen number. This will be the record key for a specimen in the SPECIMENS file. If this is not already known, the special key can be used to call up the screen for specimens in order to search for the specimen or enter a new one. The Type.type field is used to record the status of the type, which might be one of a limited number of alternatives, such as HOLO for a holotype. This field is therefore provided with data validation to make sure that only one of the right data strings can be entered. Type.cit refers to a citation in the CITATIONS file (book or journal reference, year and page number) which in return refers to a reference in the BIBLIO file. Exactly the same remarks apply to this as to the Authority field. Lastly, the Synonym.type and Synonym.of fields are to be used when the name is a synonym, and give what kind of synonym it is (e.g. partial, pro parte etc.) They can also refer to the key(s) of other record(s) in the same TAXON file to give the name of the taxon (or taxa) of which Taxon.name is a synonym. A menu appears with options for various parts of all the taxon names on it so that this is easily done by filling in some or all of the boxes. If you do not give sufficient information in the boxes to identify the other name(s), a menu appears so that the right one(s) can be selected. The screen is actually set up so that the computer 'knows' that synonym data should only be entered if the Name.type field is set for a synonym, and will object otherwise. This is yet another way in which the computer can ensure the entry of consistent data.

The procedure just described applies to filling in a new blank record. In fact, at any time, any field of the record could have been reached by moving the cursor with the arrow keys. The entry for each field could then be altered (edited) or cancelled and/or typed in again. There are then buttons which can be pressed which can be used to indicate whether the entire record is to be stored or rejected. Also, there is no need to begin with a blank record. When the screen first comes up, if the key of an existing record is typed then that record is fetched and displayed. It can then be examined or edited and stored again afterwards. The database system may allow the user to systematically examine and edit records in a process known as *browsing*. This means that the system will go from one record to the next on the press of a key, and may allow particular records to be selected or skipped according to data, and may allow the records to be visited in order. A simple program might be written to go through all the records in a file to change one or more fields, or a selection of data from one file might be added or *merged* into another. It can be seen from the above that there is in practice no clear distinction between the entry of new data and the processes of editing and updating data which is already stored, since the same programs usually do both.

2.8 Database languages

Database systems often provide one or more programming languages, which may be used to do the following:

1) define the files which are to contain the data, and the number and nature of the fields within them,

2) prepare data capture screens, menus and choice lists, manipulate the data in the files,

3) retrieve data and prepare reports, and

4) give direct one-line commands to the database system.

2.8.1 Data file definition

In most cases, the definition of files is done interactively, with the designer using the keyboard to answer a series of questions put to him by the system. The kind of information needed for these definitions is not usually regarded as a program to be executed, but is seen rather as non-procedural (non-executable) declarations. Each data file will need a name, and each field within it will need a number and/or a name. Beyond that, different database systems may have very different features. As an example, consider the file HERBARIUM as described above. In dBASEIII, the command to type as the prompt would be

CREATE HERBARIUM

and then a table will appear on the screen, with rows to fill in for each field. Each row requires the field name, its type (such as character, numeric or date), the width of the field, and, for numerics only, the number of places after the decimal point. There are only 3 or 4 properties to be supplied for each field. Appropriate entries would be:

1	Number	Numeric	5	0
2	Name	Character	80	
3	Code	Character	10	

In the case of the Name of the herbarium, 80 characters is an estimate of the longest possible name that might appear, since dBASEIII is a fixed field length system. This is rather unsatisfactory, since longer names might appear and would have to be abbreviated, whereas shorter ones will waste space.

There is a standard database language called SQL which is appearing more frequently as a feature of database systems (see below). SQL may be used interactively or not, but a suitable SQL statement equivalent to the above could be:

CREATE TABLE HERBARIUM (NUMBER DECIMAL(5) NOT NULL,
                         NAME CHAR(80) NOT NULL,
                         CODE CHAR(10) NOT NULL,
                         UNIQUE (NUMBER, CODE))

This is obviously similar to the dBASEIII version. It also implies a fixed field length. The phrase NOT NULL simply says that this field may not be empty, i.e. that it is obligatory or mandatory. The line which begins with UNIQUE states that both the Number and the Code must be different in every record.

In the Advanced Revelation system (Cosmos, 1987), the definition of a file is interactive. As this is a highly sophisticated system, there are 33 properties possible for each field, but in practice, about 6 to 10 are all that are needed. After the field name and number, there is a field type, but not in the previous sense. Fields can either be raw data, to be entered at some stage from the keyboard, or can be computed from other fields or other files. This is a variable field length system, so there is no need to specify field width, except for specifying the length of a box on the data capture screen. If the data stored is longer than the box on the screen, it simply scrolls to left or right within the box, so that a different part of the field becomes visible. There is a variety of means whereby data conversion and validation can be specified for input, and conversion for output. If the field is a date, for example, the date could be stored without any conversion so that the string of characters in the memory is just the same as the data string typed in. Alternatively, it could also be converted to a single integer before being stored, and converted back again to some suitable date format on output, and this might be different from the input format. The idea of a data type, such as character, integer, etc. for a field is optional since there are so many ways available for checking, storing and converting input data. There is a choice of different ways of expressing defaults for a field, such as having the next number in sequence, or having it the same as last time. A field can be optional or mandatory, as in SQL. There is an option to have alphabetic input text converted to upper case. It is possible to set up a help screen to be made available in conjunction with a field, so that when data capture is in progress, the user can press a special key and get an explanation of what data is expected. A very important feature is that it is possible to set up a choice menu or pop-up for any field, as required, as described above. This is a special case of a more general feature, since it is possible to set up calls to user subroutines before, during and after the entry of data in each field, and at various other points during the execution of the screen. This makes it possible to customise the system in a huge variety of ways.

2.8.2 Database processing

Database languages which can search for data, modify stored data and create reports using the data, necessarily produce executable code, and are procedural languages. The simplest alternative from the programmer's point of view is when a standard high-level programming language such as BASIC, C or PASCAL can be used. There is then no need to learn a new and special purpose programming language. Ideally, programs would refer to the database by calling subroutines from within the high-level language. If the database system programs do not cover every detailed possible requirement, then it should be possible to call user subroutines, again in the standard language, from within the database system. To put this another way, the database system is sandwiched between user code on top and more user code beneath. An example of a database system which has these features is EMPRESS (RHODNIUS, 1986). A less convenient situation is where the language provided is a special one, and only found in a particular database system.

A simple example of a database language is the programming language of dBASEIII. The following language fragment would open the file HERBARIUM, set the variable NEXT to 1, find the record which has the field NUMBER equal to 1, and store the herbarium name string from field NAME in the variable HN:

```
USE HERBARIUM
STORE 1 TO NEXT
LOCATE FOR NUMBER = NEXT
STORE NAME TO HN
```

A more sophisticated language example is Revelation-BASIC, or R/BASIC, which is special to Revelation. This is very similar to PICK BASIC, which is a feature of the PICK operating system (Taylor, 1985), which is a complete operating system designed for databases. PICK BASIC can be regarded as the standard BASIC programming language with additions for database processing. As an example, the following statements would open the HERBARIUM file, identifying it with a variable called H1, and read the record with key of 1 into the variable RECORD:

```
OPEN 'HERBARIUM' TO H1 ELSE PRINT 'error'
NEXT = 1
READ RECORD FROM H1,NEXT ELSE PRINT 'error'
```

In order to extract the name of the herbarium (which is the second field in the record) into a string variable called HN, use the statement

```
HN = RECORD<2>
```

The manner of usage of such languages as the above is such that firstly programs are written, translated or compiled with a compiling program and then executed later. An alternative approach is to provide a command language, where each statement is complete in itself, and is typed into the system on one line, causing the system to carry out that command immediately. In dBASEIII, the above program fragment could either be stored in a file and executed by a command of the form

```
DO filename
```

or typed line by line as separate commands. In order to produce a report listing the herbarium codes and names in dBASEIII it would be necessary to first set up a file which describes the desired report by the CREATE REPORT command. This is a full-screen interactive command which asks the user for details of the report that is needed. In order to carry out the report, use a command such as

```
REPORT FROM filename TO PRINT
```

On the other hand, PICK has a separate command language called ACCESS, which is mirrored in Revelation by Terminal Control Language commands (TCL for short). ACCESS deliberately imitates natural English language in order to make it easier to use. It is typically used for retrieval of data and making simple reports. As an example, to print a list of herbarium codes and names in alphabetical order of the codes, a suitable command would be:

```
LIST HERBARIUM CODE NAME BY CODE (P)
```

This LIST command names the HERBARIUM file to be used, states that the fields CODE and NAME are to be output, in that order, and that the whole is to be put into alphabetical order by CODE. The letter P in brackets means that output is to go to the printer. Revelation also has an interactive program for setting up reports corresponding to the CREATE REPORT statement of dBASEIII. Although ACCESS and PICK BASIC are distinct languages, the two can easily be combined, since any ACCESS statement can be executed within BASIC.

The HyperText language is associated with the HyperCard system (Goodman, 1987) which was first produced only for Macintosh microcomputers. HyperCard is a combination of a non-relational database system, a personal information manager and a program for creating graphics images. HyperCard is highly image oriented, and data capture and retrieval screens are presented literally as pictures, usually of file cards with data written on them as in a manual card index. This imagery is carried over into the jargon by calling records 'cards' and files 'stacks'. Unlike many other current database systems, HyperCard includes images as data, and the images can either be created internally or imported from elsewhere. HyperCard is not a relational database system, and instead it relies heavily on user-created 'links' between file records. Its strong feature is its user friendliness, but it lacks powerful indexing and sorting features. HyperText, like PICK ACCESS, superficially resembles written English, and is also related to PASCAL. It can be used both for commands and in interpreted stored programs, called 'scripts'. The scripts are activated by 'events' such as pointing with a mouse, the press of a key, or a call from another script. A program fragment equivalent to the examples given above might read

```
on MouseUp
go to stack "herbarium"
put card field id 2 into hn
```

2.8.3 Creating data capture screens

In some database systems such as the original version of dBASEIII there is no special provision for the construction of data capture screens, other than the standard editing programs, and the programmer will have to write such programs as they are needed. On the other hand, in systems such as dBASEIV, Advanced Revelation and EMPRESS there is a *fourth generation language*, or 4GL for short, for preparing data capture screens. In Revelation this 4GL is called R/DESIGN. In a regular (third generation) programming language, such as BASIC or C, the compiling program does not help the programmer to create a program, and knows nothing of the kinds of programs which might be written. A 4GL is a program which writes programs within a certain general class of programs, and in this case these are data capture programs. The broad outline of a type of data capture program has already been written and stored, and the system requests the user to give the finer details. A 4GL does not usually take the form of a written programming language, but is more often an interactive program. R/DESIGN is interactive, and initially presents a blank screen on which the programmer or designer is said to 'paint' the screen that is wanted. This means that the cursor keys are available to move a pointer around the screen so as to mark the position where each field is going to be, and the names which they are going to have. At the same time the system prompts for the entry of the other properties of fields as discussed above. During the 'painting' process, the screen looks very little different from something like that in Fig. 2.5, except that until the process is complete, the later fields are missing.

The above examples only give a few of the simpler possible ways in which a database programming language might be used. In more sophisticated applications, programs might be written to systematically alter the fields within the files, to create completely new files, or to produce complex reports. With a sophisticated system relatively little of such programming will be necessary, since the system itself will provide the means to carry out a wide range of complex manipulations. On the other hand, the more complex the system the more the effort required to learn it.

2.8.4 Structured query language

At the time of writing, there is an initiative in progress to create a standard database language for the purposes described above. This is known as Structured Query Language, or SQL for short (pronounced 'sequel'). Most relational database systems do already include SQL, or will include it in forthcoming versions. SQL is not a complete programming language in itself, unlike the other languages mentioned above, but is intended to be added to existing languages. There is nothing in the standard which insists on the manner of implementation; SQL may be a compiled or interactive language or both. As an example, in the ORACLE database system (Oracle, 1987), SQL can be embedded in various languages, although the interface to the C language is preferred. In spite of the standardisation of SQL, some authors are critical of its adequacy and its design (Date, 1987, Appendix E). One important criticism is that SQL only permits fixed-length fields and a limited set of data types, i.e. character strings, numerical values and logical (true or false).

SQL uses the terms 'row' for a record and 'column' for a field. The complete definition of all the tables or files required for an application is called a *schema*. Each table may be treated as a real (base) table in which all rows and columns are accessible, or may be treated via a more restricted *view*, where the user is only allowed to see or alter parts of the table. The data manipulation operations are called SELECT, INSERT, UPDATE and DELETE. It is fairly evident from the names of these operations as to what they do, and generally they operate simultaneously on several rows of a table at a time. Conditions involving the values of stated columns can be used to select particular rows, and the rows can be put in numerical or alphabetic order. There is an option called DISTINCT which controls whether multiple rows which contain all the same column values (as affected by a VIEW) are kept or rejected. The JOIN operation is available in order to create a new table by merging data from other tables. A number of functions are provided for performing calculations on the column data, such as COUNT, MAX (for maximum) and MIN (for minimum). It is possible to set up a list of rows from a table, i.e. a selection of rows according to some criterion, referring to something less than the complete contents of the table. This is called, somewhat confusingly, a CURSOR. A cursor is created by opening a table, selecting the required rows, and then closing the table again. Lastly, the GRANT operation is used to control user access and provide security.

2.9 Description printing

Although historically morphological descriptions were first stored in data files rather than in databases, the distinction is not really significant. At first sight, it might seem strange to use a computer to generate printed descriptions, when much descriptive information is initially in printed form. However, as more and more descriptive data is converted to computerised form, it becomes more natural to collect such data via some kind of data capture screen, store it in some format such as DELTA, (p. 111) and then convert it by suitable programs into whatever form is needed. The two obvious uses of printed descriptions are firstly, for the proof-reading of the factual accuracy of descriptive data stored in computers, and secondly, as a preliminary to the word processing of descriptions for publication. Morse (1974) described a program which printed simple descriptions, with one character per line. A more recent description printing program will be described here, based on DELTA format. DELTA data is converted to printed descriptions in conventional language with sentences, paragraphs, punctuation and summaries of characters of taxonomic groups. Full allowance is made for character variation, character dependencies, the elimination of repetitive phrases, and the expression of numerical characters. An earlier version of this program is described by Pankhurst (1978b).

An example of the program output is shown in Fig. 2.7. The program accepts additional data which defines which characters are to be used and in what order, and how they are to be arranged in sentences and paragraphs. The way in which the characters and states are defined in words in DELTA is critical to the style of the resulting text, and a little thought needs to be given to this. Some users prefer to have more than one version of the character descriptions containing different wordings for essentially the same descriptive data, according to the purpose for whicn the characters are to be used. If a sequence of characters is assigned to a sentence, then it will be assumed that the characters can all be given the same name, e.g. characters 11 and 12 in the figure are put into the same sentence, and so the sentence 'leaves compound, leaves digitate' is simplified to 'leaves compound, digitate'. If the name string 'leaves' had not been the same in both characters, a warning message would have appeared. The distinction between sequential and non-sequential multistate characters is important in descriptions, since variation in sequential characters can be abbreviated, e.g. 'wings small, or medium, or large' will be shortened to 'wings small to large', whereas non-sequential characters have to be spelt out in full, with 'or' preceding the alternative states. If successive states have a phrase in common, like 'leaves shorter than stem, or as long as stem', this will be shortened to 'leaves shorter than, or as long as stem'. Dependent characters may give rise to a special situation, if the controlling character varies, e.g. 'wings absent or present, wings yellow' meaning yellow if present, can be printed by the program as 'wings absent, or present and yellow', provided that they are put into the same sentence in the

RUBUS in CENTRAL AMERICA   Revised 8.1986

(11) Leaves usually compound. (26) Inflorescence with 1 to 200 flowers. (29) Inflorescence axis glandular hairs 0.1 to 6.0mm. (30) Inflorescence axis non-glandular bristles usually absent. (32) Petals 0.3 to 2.5 cm. (35) Sepals 0.3 to 3.0 cm. (39) Fruit 0.4 to 3.5 cm. (42) Drupelets 4 to 200.

1.   Adenotrichus
(1) Stem prostrate or ascending, (2) biennial, (3) not pruinose. (46) Stipules linear. (4) Stem simple hairs numerous. (5) Stem glandular hairs numerous. (7) Stem non-glandular bristles absent. (8) Stem prickles fairly many, (9) straight and curved, (10) about equal stem width.
(11) Leaves compound, (12) digitate. (13) Leaves not coriaceous, (14) paler green below. (15) Leaves with some simple hairs above, (16) with some simple hairs below, (17) more numerous on veins.
(19) Leaflets elliptic or lanceolate, (20) rounded at base, (21) emarginate. (22) Leaflets simply serrate or biserrate, (23) regularly serrate. (24) Leaflet teeth under 1mm. (18) Leaflet veins below not prominent.
(44) Flowering hermaphrodite. (25) Inflorescence compound. (26) Inflorescence with 30 to 90 flowers. (27) Inflorescence axis simple hairs numerous. (28) Inflorescence axis glandular hairs numerous, (29) 0.2 to 6.0mm, (45) unequal. (30) Inflorescence axis non-glandular bristles absent. (31) Inflorescence axis prickles few.
(34) Petals white or pink, (32) 0.4 to 1.0 cm, (33) 1–2 times sepals. (35) Sepals 0.4 to 0.7 cm, (36) patent in fruit.
(38) Fruit ovoid, (39) 0.5 to 1.0 cm. (42) Drupelets 15 to 40, (41) glabrous.

Fig. 2.7   Computer generated description of part of genus *Rubus*.

right order. As options, comments from the DELTA data can also be printed, and the character numbers can be added to the output, as in Fig. 2.7.

It is possible to obtain character summaries when, for example, the taxa are members of a genus which is divided into subgenera. As part of the additional data, the user can divide the taxa into groups with titles, and then each group will have a character summary printed. This will list all characters which are constant within the group, and also those which occur most frequently with the adverb 'usually' added, as happens with character 30 in the figure. Here 'usually' means in X% or more cases, where X may be set to, say, 80%. In this way, accurate descriptions of higher level taxa may be obtained. Quantitative characters are summarised so as to give a range of the lowest and highest values in the group.

Dallwitz (1984) describes another description printing program based on DELTA, to which automatic typesetting options have been added. This allows the taxonomist to go much further towards creating the finished text for his publications, but typesetting by computer is not yet standardised for general use, and the production of camera-ready copy by means of one of the popular desktop publishing packages is an attractive alternative. Skov (1989a) describes a description printing option which is genuinely integrated with a database which forms part of his floristic database based on the HyperCard database system.

2.10 Applications

2.10.1 Existing single-purpose taxonomic databases

Examples are discussed according to the five types of taxonomic data as listed above (p. 12). The earliest database systems tended to concentrate on one kind of data only, whereas in recent years there has been a move to create general-purpose databases with different kinds of data linked together.

1)   A review of curatorial databases for plants is given by Pankhurst (1984). Of the nine systems discussed there, two have been selected for further comment. The oldest surviving curatorial database system for plants is undoubtedly the Flora of Veracruz project (Gómez-Pompa and Nevling, 1973; Gómez-Pompa *et al.*, 1984) which was initiated in the mid-1960s. In view of rapid destruction of tropical forests and the lack of detailed knowledge of them, it is also of great importance for the fact that it is both a database for tropical plants and situated in the tropics. The initial effort was concentrated on creating a database of specimen labels, and this was maintained for a new but rapidly growing herbarium at Jalapa, currently comprising over 60 000 specimens. At first, about 60 data fields were specified for each label, but this was found to be impractical and was later reduced to about 30 (Fig. 2.6). One of the early products of the database was a checklist of species names for the area, which was indispensable as a reference. A novel product of the database was the index to medicinal plants and their uses (del Amo, 1979). The Flora of Veracruz project began to consider morphological character data at an early stage, and has made considerable use of DELTA programs (Gómez-Pompa *et al.*, 1984), especially for a key to plant families of the region. Computerised maps of plant distribution and of other geographical factors have been produced, and the exploitation of colour graphics images in video or digital form is being actively pursued.

The Smithsonian Institution in Washington also began to catalogue its collections by computer at an early date, i.e. in the late 1960s. Over the museum as a whole there are currently more than 3 million specimen records stored on databases. Of these, the department of vertebrate zoology at over 900 000 has the most records. The botanical records stand at about 440 000, of which over 86 000 comprise a register of type specimens. Various different database systems are in use, including dBASEIII, an IBM system called INQUIRE, and the SELGEM system (Creighton and Crockett, 1971), which was developed within the institution. SELGEM was designed to allow for variable length fields, and has a hierachical (not relational) data structure. The SELGEM retrieval commands are rather like those of the ACCESS language in PICK (see above). Abbott *et al.* (1985, Chapter 12) describe an application of SELGEM.

2)   *The Atlas of the British Flora* (Perring and Walters, 1962) was probably the first large-scale computerised species mapping project, and contains dot maps for about 1 700 plants, Fig 2.8. Whilst the original maps were produced by a punched card system which has long been obsolete, the records have since been transferred to an ORACLE database system at the Biological Records Centre of the Institute of Terrestrial Ecology. There are currently about 4.4 million records held on minicomputers. Data has been collected and added to the system for a period of over thirty years, and now covers over 9 000 species of animals and plants.

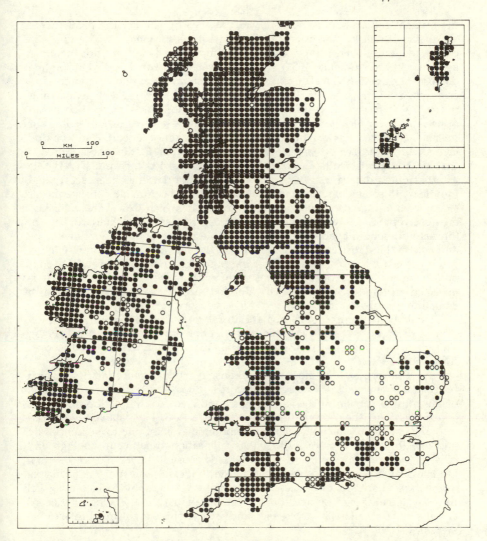

Fig. 2.8 Distribution map of *Drosera rotundifolia* in the British Isles (Courtesy of The Biological Records Centre).

A different example of mapping from a database is provided by the *Flora of Warwickshire* (Cadbury *et al.*, 1971). In this case there are over 700 maps of species distribution within one county, and with habitat types shown by special symbols.

3) The Index Kewensis is the principal reference for botanical nomenclature. It was originally published in book form (1893), and has been kept more or less up to date with a series of supplements. It includes the scientific names of species and genera of flowering plants with the author and place of publication, and with some information on the geographical distribution. In

the original volumes an assessment was made as to whether the names were acceptable or not, but this was abandoned with the supplements. Many of the earlier references were simply compiled without checking, and are therefore apt to be in error (Meikle, 1971). The Index has been converted to an on-line database using the STATUS text retrieval system on a minicomputer, and currently contains over 940 000 records, including over 42 000 genera and over 860 000 species (Lucas,1989). Interestingly, the data was captured by an optical character recognition process, followed by extensive proof-reading for misread characters. Apart from some relatively minor uncorrected copying errors, the database is therefore identical in content to the publication, so that all its existing faults and virtues have been carried forward. STATUS is a text-oriented database system, and although the data has been segregated into fields to some degree, some of these have not been made consistent. For example, the references to books and journals in which taxa were published are just reproduced verbatim, without cross reference to standard lists of journal and book title abbreviations. The same is true of author abbreviations and geographical distribution. In spite of these qualifications, the on-line Index Kewensis is extremely useful as a starting point for a revision of a plant group, and is much more convenient for searching than the printed version. It is expected that Index Kewensis will soon be made more widely available in computer-readable form.

A zoological example of a nomenclatural (and bibliographic) publication from a database was the catalogue of Hymenoptera (Krombein *et al.*, 1974). This database was created using the SELGEM system at the Smithsonian Institution.

4)   The largest and most comprehensive bibliographic database which covers taxonomy is the Zoological Record, (BIOSIS, 1985). The publication of the printed version of the Record has continued for over a hundred years (since 1865), and the computerised version since 1978. The database is divided into 27 sections of which 25 relate to taxonomic groups, one to nomenclature and one for general topics. Over 6 000 publications relating to zoology and palaeontology are covered, and the on-line database has over 600 000 records. On-line searches are aided by a sophisticated indexing scheme. The principal indices are to authors of articles, subject matter, geography, palaeontological time, systematics and source (titles of publications). The Zoological Record On-line is internationally accessible, and is a sophisticated and professional system.

A botanical database equivalent to the Zoological Record is the Kew Record, although it is considerably smaller and of much more recent origin. It is implemented in the same way as the Index Kewensis (see above). A smaller example of a bibliographic database, used by a small research group studying Crustacea, is described by Sieg (1984). For the creation of data dictionaries for abbreviations of titles of books and journals, botanists can use the *Taxonomic Literature 2* (TL2 for short, Stafleu and Cowan, 1976-1988) and *B-P-H* (Lawrence *et al.*, 1968), respectively, both of which are in the process of being turned into databases.

5)   There are numerous DELTA data sets in existence which contain data on morphological and other characters. It is arguable as to whether these are databases in the strict sense, but the largest of them is impressive. The data on grass genera of the world by Watson and Dallwitz (1988) covers 765 taxa with 469 characters. Earlier versions of this publication included

the descriptions in print as well as extensive identification keys derived by DELTA programs, but now the data is distributed only by floppy disc with an accompanying identification program with some retrieval features (INTKEY, p. 124). The printed publication is now mostly devoted to character illustrations. Winfield and Green (1984) describe a database of plant morphology which is not applied to species but to cultivars. The problem here is to establish the individuality of new commercial varieties of crop plants. This sytem does not use DELTA.

Other special-purpose databases exist which do not fall into the above categories. One of these is a database for the description of vegetation (Nimis *et al.*, 1984), and there are several databases for phytochemistry (Charlwood *et al.*, 1984, and Babaç and Bisby, 1984). Mackinder (1984) describes a database for species conservation. It is unlikely that these few examples cover all the possibilities.

2.10.2 Existing general-purpose taxonomic databases

One example of a general-purpose database has already been described in detail above (Section 2.6). A selection of other important projects will now be discussed.

PRECIS (the Pretoria National Herbarium Computerised Information System) is another general-purpose botanical database, and one of the first to be established (Morris, 1974). Its design and content is roughly similar to that of the TROPICOS system (see below). Historically, it began as a specimen-based system, and specimen-PRECIS contains all the data from labels in the herbarium collection, currently about 660 000 (Russell and Arnold, 1989). The fact that this data is complete and is kept up to date is most important, as it permits a very wide range of useful reports to be produced. These include a variety of sorted lists of specimens, area checklists, collection inventory, lists of specimens according to collectors, distribution maps of species and maps of collecting intensity. This information is all the more valuable since South Africa happens to have one of the richest temperate floras in the world, and no complete national flora has been published. The nomenclatural part of PRECIS is in two parts, actually called taxon-PRECIS and nomenclatural-PRECIS. Taxon-PRECIS began as a list of all accepted species names with authors, to which was added recent synonyms and literature references, and subsequently various kinds of taxon-oriented data, very much the same as the 'common knowledge' data of ILDIS (see below). Where appropriate, however, (as for geographical distribution) this data was compiled from specimen-PRECIS. Nomenclatural-PRECIS has species names with complete synonymy and literature references, but is not complete, except for two large families which were entered on a trial basis. The three components of PRECIS discussed so far are all implemented on a mainframe computer. The last component, curatorial-PRECIS, is based on a microcomputer network, and handles the preparation of labels for new material and is used for loans management. Among the useful products are lists of determinations, lists of species for loans and files of mailing addresses. A list of accepted and accurately spelt taxon names from the mainframe part of PRECIS is used here to make sure that all names on labels and in lists are correct. It is interesting to read in the most recent account of PRECIS (Russell and Arnold, 1989) of the managerial problems experienced over the years.

TROPICOS is a general-purpose botanical taxonomic database at the Missouri Botanical Garden (Crosby and Magill, 1989). It runs under the PICK operating system on a special-purpose mini-computer, and is programmed in the PICK BASIC language (see p. 27). It is therefore generally incompatible with other systems, but data can be imported and exported to IBM/PC compatible microcomputers. The PC version is known as pcTROPICOS, and uses the Revelation database system (p. 26). TROPICOS is divided into different sections for vascular plants and mosses, and contains data relating to both specimens and to taxa. At the time of writing, TROPICOS contains data on over 430 000 plant names and over 100 000 types.

The principal files within TROPICOS are those for nomenclature, bibliography, geographical distribution and specimens. The nomenclature file contains scientific and vernacular names and refers to the bibliography file for the publication references and citations and to a specimen file for the types. The data from the computerised *Index Nominum Genericorum* (ING, Farr *et al.*, 1979) was used as a basis for the generic names. Synonymy has been included, and the database stores references to those bibliographic entries that accept or reject each name. There is a separate file for author name abbreviations. The bibliography is based on the standard lists of the *B-P-H* (1968) and *Taxonomic Literature 2* (TL2 for short, Stafleu and Cowan, 1976-1988) as well as additions. It currently contains about 15 000 references. Data on geographical distribution can be stored at the level of country, state and county (or equivalents) and the records of plant distribution are based on published literature or on label data from specimen files. The geographical scheme is complete to the level of state (province) for the New World. There are three separate files for specimens: for types, herbarium label data for new material, and exsiccatae (existing herbarium specimens which are not types). The first two of these files contain specialised data which is not required for most specimens, but their other information can be moved into the exsiccatae file in order to provide a single file for all specimens. TROPICOS can be used for the entry and printing of labels for new material, and in the process, scientific names are checked for accuracy against the existing names stored on file. The system can also be used for the management of loans. Apart from the main files just described, there are additional files for other data, such as a chromosome number file and a plant uses file. There is a small file of morphological descriptive data. Characters are stored in coded form, as in DELTA, and can be sorted and searched as an aid to keymaking. Descriptions in the form of word-processable text can be generated. Work is underway to install an interface to DELTA software for use in floristic projects. TROPICOS is being used for the flora of North America and for the English language version of the flora of China.

A major floristic database is that for the *Flora Europaea* (Tutin *et al.*, 1964-80). The computerised database was created after the flora had been published (Heywood *et al.*, 1984) and essentially contains the same factual information as the publication, but not including the descriptions and keys. However, while the database was being built, errors and inconsistencies in the published version were found and removed. The main data categories are the nomenclature with synonymy, geographical distribution within and outside Europe, the literature references, and cytology. The data was stored under the ORACLE database system (Oracle, 1987), using both mainframe and microcomputer versions. The first product from the Flora Europaea database was a checklist of European pteridophytes (Derrick *et al.*, 1987). This database has now been converted to Advanced Revelation.

The Vicieae database (Adey *et al.*, 1984) was an early attempt to create a monographic database and involved about 400 taxa. Unlike many other databases described here, it was intentionally oriented towards users of taxonomic information, rather than just for taxonomists themselves. It was a taxon-based system, with data on nomenclature, including synonymy, geographical distribution, morphology and phytochemistry (Babaç and Bisby, 1984) but without a bibliography and without any specimen data. The morphological data was processed by DELTA programs to produce keys and descriptions. The Vicieae database acted as a pilot project for the much more comprehensive International Legume Database and Information Service (ILDIS, 1988) which followed it.

The ILDIS database is a database to record the diversity of the legume family of plants (Leguminosae or Fabaceae). It is based on a world checklist of accepted names, and is intended to provide data on crops, products, conservation and distribution as well as links to other kinds of information and expertise. It is a taxon-based system, and will not contain any information about specimens. ILDIS is planned as not only a database but also as an information service to a wide range of users of data about legumes. It has a solid taxonomic basis but will not be primarily a database for taxonomists.

The first phase of ILDIS is creating a complete world list of around 15 000 accepted scientific names for legumes with synonymy and includes a judgement about which names are accepted and which are not. This is an innovation, since neither in this nor in any other large plant family has there ever been any international consensus on the subject before. However, there will not be any information stored about types or type specimens. Geographical distribution data about these taxa is stored at continent, country and state levels. The 'common knowledge' section includes data on vernacular names, life form, vegetation types, conservation status, and uses, plus references to published descriptions, illustrations and maps. The standards for definition of world geographical areas and conservation status will be those laid down by the TDWG organisation (p. 190). The ALICE software (see below) is being used to capture data for this first phase.

The first version of the ALICE system (Allkin and Winfield, 1989) was developed for use with the ILDIS database, but is not restricted to that. ALICE is a generalised species diversity database system. It was written in the dBASE language, first as a dBASEII application and later in dBASEIII, and is therefore a fixed field length system. It is a taxon-based system, and only later versions have any provision for data on specimens. It has a sophisticated nomenclature section, which deals intelligently with synonyms, homonyms and taxa at different taxonomic levels. Geographical distribution data are held at various levels, but what these levels are may be specified by the user. For example, in ILDIS, three levels are used, namely continent, country and province. ALICE makes sense of distributional information at the different levels, e.g. if a plant is recorded in New York, then it is also recorded for the U.S.A. There is a bibliography section for referring to publications and other data sources. Care has been taken in the system design to be sure that, where the user thinks appropriate, the source of any data can be traced, so that it is

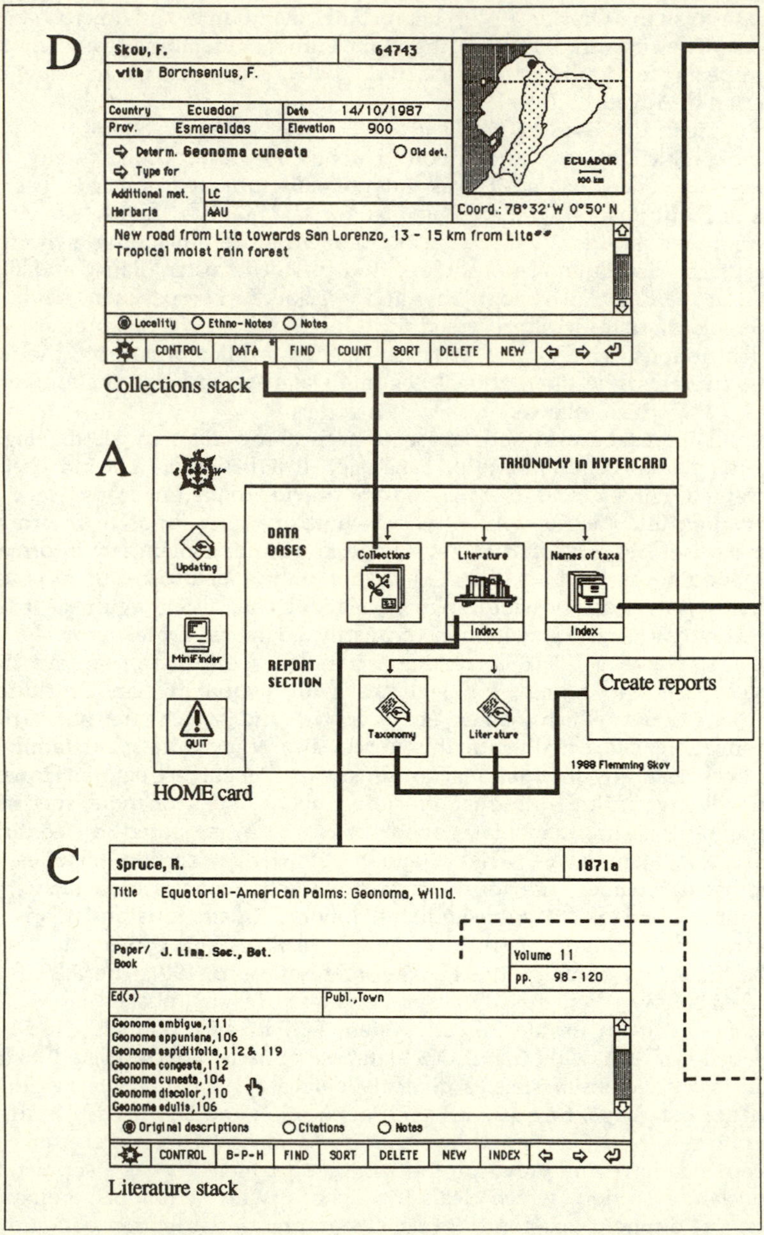

Fig. 2.9   Screens from HyperTaxonomy, (after Skov).

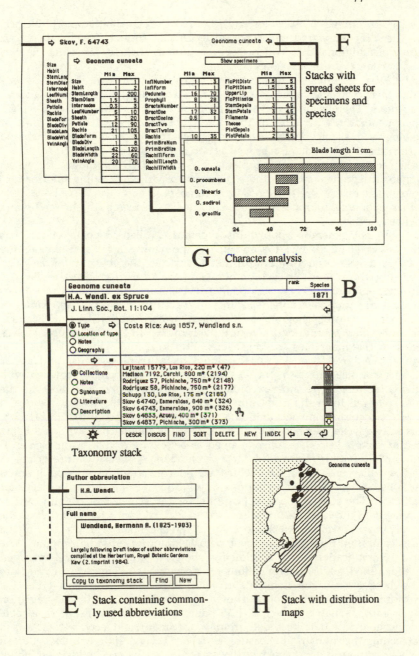

F Stacks with spread sheets for specimens and species

G Character analysis

Taxonomy stack **B**

E Stack containing commonly used abbreviations

H Stack with distribution maps

possible to retrieve the basis for any recorded fact. Qualitative morphological characters can be stored and exported to DELTA format. Finally, there is a variety of additional data which can be recorded, such as vernacular names, uses, habitat, and free text notes.

ALICE has a number of database system features of its own. The users may define their own qualitative characters and states, and other general-purpose descriptors. There is an ALICE query program for data retrieval and an ALICE report generator. There are utilities for import and export of data and for merging and slicing databases. The applications of ALICE have included zoological and ethnobotanical as well as botanical projects.

The second phase of ILDIS is planned to include a wide range of practical data about legumes, such as the commercial products, breeding information, ecology, chemistry and chromosome numbers. There will also be a little further taxonomic information about intermediate names in the hierarchy and brief descriptions.

An original general-purpose floristic database called HyperTaxonomy has been designed by Skov (1989a and b). As the name suggests, it exploits the HyperCard system on a Macintosh microcomputer (see above), and has been applied by the author to a revision of a genus of palms from Ecuador. Fig. 2.9 illustrates some of the HyperTaxonomy screens. There are currently seven files ('stacks') covering collections (specimens), literature (bibliography), names of taxa (nomenclature), geographical distribution, abbreviations for publications and author names, and morphological descriptions. In Fig. 2.9, screen A gives access to the main files for collections, literature and names of taxa. The diagrams in boxes (icons) can be pointed to by using a mouse and act as 'buttons' for selecting different files. The screens are liberally provided with buttons for moving to other records or files of various kinds. These are the 'links' referred to in the discussion of HyperCard (p. 28). Screen B shows a record containing nomenclatural data, with content similar to that in Fig. 2.5. This screen has a number of options, and at the moment shown, was being used to make a list of specimens named as belonging to that taxon. Screen C shows bibliographic information for a publication. A special feature of this is the box which lists all the taxa which are referred to within this publication. These names can be used as buttons to jump to the nomenclatural detail for that taxon. The specimen record ('card') shown in screen D is roughly similar in content to the label already discussed in Fig. 2.1, with the addition of the country map which shows the location of the specimen. The position of the dot is computed from the coordinate data field and inserted by program. The current identification of the specimen is shown in a box, but if the specimen is re-identified, older determinations are remembered. The taxon names are cross-checked with the nomenclature file. If the specimen is a type, the taxon for which it is a type is shown. Screen E contains the abbreviation for an author's name as well as the name in full. Screen F shows a table of morphological data recorded from a specimen, and screen G shows a plot comparing numerical measurements for several different taxa. Screen H shows a map for a taxon which was computed by combining data about determined specimens and taxon names.

As with any database system, HyperTaxonomy's files can be used to search for and retrieve any combination of stored data. A significant part of the taxonomic process which is provided is the means to combine tabulated morphological descriptions from specimens into a description of a taxon, and to convert this to text with a description-writing program. This data can also be output in DELTA format so that the various DELTA programs for key construction can be applied to it. The resulting text still needs some manual editing before it is suitable for publication. Another feature of the system is a simple interactive identification program, which performs step-by-step elimination of taxa based on the characters of an unknown specimen. Four different kinds of data lists can be produced by HyperTaxonomy, and these include lists of specimens seen, lists of miscellaneous notes from specimen labels, lists of synonyms and lists of literature references. The automatic production of such data in word processor form contributes considerably to the routine work of preparing a taxonomic monograph.

2.10.3 Further data on taxa

There are of course no hard and fast rules as to what data is or is not appropriate for databases. The discussion given above concerns databases for taxonomic purposes, but there are many other wider categories of information which, while they still need to be taxonomically based, are of interest to a wider audience. The following types of information are actually or potentially useful, but it does not follow that the data is normally available in any convenient form. This is particularly true of image data (marked with asterisks).

(1) The most frequently published types of data:
– descriptions of the gross morphology of the taxa,
– identification keys, mature specimens only,
– nomenclature, the scientific plant names and their authors,
– synopsis, a summary of the classification in use,
– bibliography, principal titles,
– geographical distribution, often in terms of subdivisions such as states or counties,
– ecological data, such as altitude range, habitat, predators, associated taxa etc.,
– glossary of descriptive terms used, diagrams* of morphological characters,
– uses of taxa, e.g. for food, as medicine, whether poisonous,
– evolutionary speculations about the origins of the taxa.

(2) Less frequently published types of data:
– bibliography of where taxa are published, and comprehensive bibliography in general,
– references to other descriptions and where illustrations are published,
– illustrations* of whole organisms, monochrome or coloured line drawings or photos,
– type specimen data, especially the location of specimens,
– alternative classifications,
– maps* of taxon distributions,
– descriptions and photos* of habitat,
– biological data: biotic factors, mycorrhiza, insect/animal relationships, pathology, genetics, population dynamics, behaviour, pollination mechanisms.

– biography: history of collectors in the region, portraits*,
– detailed photos* of morphological characters, e.g. genitalia of insects; micrographs or electron micrographs* of, e.g. pollen, seeds, chromosomes,
– notes of which specimens were examined,
– regional geography: climate, geology and human populations, with maps*,
– ethnology: traditional uses and folklore,
– gazetteers: index of place names and geographical locations.
(3) Least frequently published types of data:
– descriptions of juveniles, detailed leaf anatomy, pollen etc.,
– identification keys to juveniles or detached parts,
– field records of taxa in localities, especially for nature reserves,
– label data from preserved specimens,
– records of species in botanical or zoological gardens or parks, seed banks, germplasm collections,
– images* of preserved specimens, especially types (sometimes available as microfiche) and important historical material,
– published maps*, aerial and land satellite photos*,
– images* of selected pages from rare books, notebooks of important collectors and other manuscripts,
– conservation data: status, threats,
– data on cultivation or husbandry, management of living collections,
– biochemical data,
– anything about related fossils,
– videos* or movie films* of habitats, insect or animal behaviour.

An independent and very detailed list of the information that a floristic database could or should contain, and the potential uses and users of such data, are given in relation to the flora of North America project by Morin *et al.* (1989).

2.10.4 Future impact of databases on taxonomy

Although textual and numerical data has so far dominated the discussion of taxon databases, it is clear that technology will shortly become available which will enable image data to be included in databases, and that this will have an enormous impact, especially with the use of colour. A video or digital image is not necessarily a complex object from the point of view of a database system. The minimum representation of an image would simply be the address (or file name) of where it is stored, since the database need not necessarily hold any other data about the image. Viewed thus, an image data field is no more complex than a field representing, say, a person's name, apart from the fact that it requires considerable storage space. Other data relating to the image, such as the name of the subject, when and where it was taken, and where other related images are to be found, can be treated as conventional database fields. The power of such a system will derive from the ability to recall images as the result of a retrieval request, based on the related data, which will be a statement about what kind of image(s) are wanted. In addition to this, the image when viewed will contain information which will be perceived by the viewer, and this may in turn be entered into the database as new factual information. In other words, it will be useful to store data on the contents and structure of the images as well as the images themselves. It is also possible for fresh images to be created on the basis of factual and/or image information already stored, such as the drawing of maps. It will therefore be very useful to provide the means not merely to retrieve data and images already present, but to permit the users to add their own data and images to their copy of the database, just as a word processor's spelling checker may allow you to create your own personal dictionary. In general, a user may want to transform any kind of information already present into new data. This might include

- generating maps or tree diagrams,
- measuring sizes and shapes of organs from preserved specimens or drawings and turning these into morphological descriptions,
- cutting, rotating, scaling and recolouring video images into digital images for use in identification programs, or
- editing of text and images for output to desktop publishing systems.

While images may be initially thought of as flat, two-dimensional pictures, there may be some need to process three-dimensional images, or construct 3-D images from a succession of 2-D images. This might be applied to subjects such as pollen grains, spores, or Protozoa; to 3-D growth patterns in inflorescences or trees, or to multidimensional output from principal coordinate analysis.

3

Classification

3.1 Introduction

The term *classification* refers to the placing of objects in groups in such a way that the members of the groups bear a closer relationship to other members of the same group than they do to members of other groups. The process of forming groups may be called *grouping* or *clustering*. It is quite possible that a useful classification cannot be made with a given set of data, if the data has no structure. Even if that were the case, there is normally nothing to actually prevent clustering methods being applied to the data; what happens is that the results are meaningless. When a classification has been created with a set of data, one may either say that the structure of the data has been 'uncovered', or else that all that has happened is that a convenient manner of summarising the data has been found, and that the classification has simply been 'imposed'. There is often no experimental evidence which will enable these two philosophies to be distinguished. The theory and methods of classification are applied to a wide variety of different kinds of objects; animate or inanimate, actual or conceptual. If the objects classified are biological taxa, then we have a biological classification. Extensive classifications of plants and animals do of course already exist, and will be found in textbooks of botany and zoology. The details of these will not be discussed here. The term *relationship* can mean various different things, and is a source of confusion in the literature. When biologists speak of relationships between organisms, they might mean

1) *phenetic* relationships, based on a comparison of physical characters (morphology) or the phenotype. The *phenotype* is the set of characters of the present-day living organism. To this might be added breeding relationships and ecological relationships.

2) *phylogenetic* or *cladistic* relationships, based on theories of the evolutionary history of organisms, or

3) *genetic* relationships, based on the genetic constitution of organisms, or even actual knowledge of the molecular sequences in DNA and RNA (genomic relationships).

Each of these types of relationship can be interpreted in greater detail, and will in general be different for any given group of organisms (see below).

Once a classification has been created, names are invented to give to each of the different groups. Taxonomic *nomenclature* is a subject in its own right, and will not be pursued further here. There are rule books which govern the use of taxonomic names. For further information, see a textbook of taxonomy such as Davis and Heywood (1963), Lawrence (1951), or Mayr (1969).

A little definition is required when speaking of the objects which are being classified. In order not to prejudice the issue in advance by assuming that groups actually exist, and to avoid assuming that these should have any particular taxonomic rank, the phrase *operational taxonomic unit* (or OTU for short) is often used for the objects under study. Since the phrase is ugly, and its abbreviation mystifying, OTUs will simply be referred to as 'objects'. In the biological context, these objects might be specimens, species or other taxa.

Classifications are fundamental, not only to biology, but to the whole of human language. The use of concrete nouns in language depends on having an agreed classification of objects, as well as having agreed names for them. The use of a simple notion in speech such as 'table' depends on both the speaker and the listeners knowing what tables are like, and all agreeing on what they are to be called. This is very well illustrated in the famous passage in Lewis Carroll's *Through the Looking Glass* where Alice goes into the wood where things have no names, and finds that it becomes impossible to hold a conversation (see title pages). Schemes of classification are therefore vital to biology as a reference system; a means to define what plants or animals are being studied. This reference system also makes it possible to search the literature and to retrieve all kinds of information about organisms.

Biological classifications are, unfortunately, subject to change with time. This may be because new data are discovered about organisms which need to be taken into account, such as the discovery of new species, or the collection of new kinds of data about known species. It may also be because better classifications have been found, although there is a risk that what are claimed to be better classifications may be based on nothing more than subjective personal opinion. Names may also change merely because of the application of the rules of nomenclature. Needless to say, the usefulness of classifications depends in part on their *stability*, and so biological classifications ought not to be changed unnecessarily. Those who need to use taxonomic information but who are not taxonomists often complain about apparently needless name changes. However, since there are so many species still to be discovered, especially in the tropics, some of the root causes of instability can scarcely be avoided. There is in fact a continuous cycle in which the discovery of new information leads to the creation of new classifications (see Section 5.9).

Even in view of the above, what can be done to make sure that classifications are stable? Firstly, when selecting the initial set of objects before trying to form groups, all the relevant objects must be included. Secondly, all the significant characters of the objects and all their variations must be included in the study. In the language of statistics, first find a truly representative sample of the population, and then measure all the variables. These requirements are not easy to satisfy. When selecting a group of organisms to classify, the characters of those organisms must be examined in order to decide whether each organism 'belongs' to the single complete starting group, or whether it does not. In other words, it is difficult to avoid circular reasoning. When choosing an initial group, there is a risk of choosing just those organisms which will agree with the patterns which one hopes to find. This is not as bad as it sounds; there does exist one finite group from which nothing is excluded, i.e. the group of all living organisms. We are certain that there are many species which have not been discovered, and in any case, that group is too large to handle with any known methods. How can we be reasonably confident that small selections from this global group are 'proper' subsets? One observation which is reassuring is that it is possible to find groups that have gaps between them. The diagram in Fig. 5.6 shows groups limited by circles. At least two of these circles have some space between them in which very few or no objects occur. Some groups have been studied for so long and in such detail that there is little chance that further unknown wild species are going to be found, e.g. birds. Lastly, the purpose for which the classification is being made may of itself define the initial group members, e.g. a classification of cultivars of some crop.

It is harder to know whether all the character variation has been included. During the current century, many new kinds of characters and ways of measuring them have been discovered, all of which provide new ways of gathering character data about organisms, e.g. cytology and electron micros- copy, to mention just two. Consequently, there is always the hope, and the risk, that new kinds of characters are going to be found in the future. It is quite clear that selecting random sets of characters out of a larger set, or sets of characters which are too small, can distort the resulting classification (Farris, 1979; Davies, 1981). This is because some characters carry more infor- mation about the objects than others do, and if some of the information-rich characters are omitted, then there is bound to be distortion. This will be discussed in more detail below. There is another possible cause of instability, which is the effect of errors in observing characters. This, however, can be minimised by repeating and cross-checking the observations on characters.

Another requirement which is sometimes placed on classifications is that they should be *predictive*. There is considerable confusion about this since the term predictivity has been used with at least four different meanings:

1)   Given that we know that a specimen is a member of a group within some existing classification based on some set of characters, we can then say what states those characters are going to have. This is not prediction; it is just information retrieval.

2)   Given a specimen of something new, such as a new species from a known genus, then we can predict what its characters are going to be. In order to recognise this specimen as a member of the existing genus, we must have used some of its characters in the identification process in order to assign it to the genus. Those characters have not been predicted, but just observed. Other characters which have not so far been looked at might be predictable.

3)   Given a group in an existing classification based on known characters, then we may be able to predict the distribution of states of other characters which have not so far been examined, which might be correlated with the states of known characters. If the original characters in our classification were determined by a degree of genetic make up which is common to all members of the group, then we can expect some of the new characters to be determined in this way also.

4)   A classification is supposed to put objects into groups in such a way that the members of each group are closer to each other than they are to the members of other groups. We can try to measure this internal group consistency by looking at the states of each character within a group. Suppose that out of 10 taxa in a group, a character has one state for 7 taxa

and another for the other 3. This character is then 70% constant within the group. A similar score can be made for other characters in the group and averaged out, and repeated for other groups. This gives a measure of average consistency of groups, and is a measure of predictivity (Sneath and Hansell, 1985). Sneath and Hansell show mathematically that this particular kind of predictivity is maximised by an unweighted average link clustering method, or if weighted, to a sum of squares clustering (p.57). Gower's method of maximal predictive classification (Gower, 1974) approaches the problem in another way (p.65). In contrast, various authors such as Mayr (1969) claim that (weighted) phylogenetic classifications will have the best predictive properties, but give no mathematical justification. If this claim were investigated numerically, one might expect to find that phylogenetic classifications do also have quite a high predictive value.

Yet another desirable property of a method of classification is its *objectivity*. This implies that it should be possible for an independent worker, given the same organisms and the same character sets, to follow a standard method and arrive at the same results. If not, then presumably either mistakes have been made or the method is somehow unsound. In practice, different and rival classifications for a given set of organisms often exist, whose relative merits are disputed. Scientists from disciplines other than biological taxonomy might be surprised on reading this; objectivity is a vital property of the scientific method in general, so what is there to dispute about? There is, however, a good deal of disagreement among taxonomists as to what kind of classifications should be created, what the purposes of classifications are to be, and how they should be achieved. Notice that objectivity is required, not merely in taxonomic procedures as they are carried out, but in the formulation of the rules for those procedures as well.

Classifications differ in detail according to the purpose for which they are intended. Some examples should make this clear. The familiar and non-scientific classification of crop plants into fruits and vegetables concentrates on the utility of the plants, how they are grown, and what part of the plant is consumed. The beetroot and the carrot are both seen as root vegetables, although taxonomically one belongs to the family Chenopodiaceae and the other to the Umbelliferae. The raspberry and the apple are seen as soft and hard fruits, respectively, but they both belong to the same family, Rosaceae. Classifications may differ according to whether they are intended to correspond to evolutionary history, or not. This is because of the occurrence of divergence and convergence. *Divergence* is the situation where taxa are closely related by ancestry but have evolved rapidly at some stage and have become physically rather different from one another. In other words, their ancestral relationship is closer than their phenetic relationship. *Convergence* is the opposite, where taxa whose ancestral relationship is rather distant have evolved in such a way, perhaps as adaptations to the same rigorous environment, that they have acquired more similar characters and their phenetic relationship is rather closer. Notice that divergence and convergence normally only affect some characters of taxa, rather than all of them. If either of these phenomena affected all characters equally then they would be impossible to detect, since there would be no evidence remaining of the 'true' relationships of the taxa concerned. If convergence has occurred, then a phylogenetic classification will associate taxa rather less closely than will a phenetic classification. Likewise, if there has been divergence, a phylogenetic classification will associate taxa more closely than a phenetic one. Of course, if there has been neither convergence or divergence, then there may be no difference at all. In general, a phylogenetic classification will be better at showing the supposed ancestral relationships, and a phenetic classification will better represent the characters of current-day organisms. It needs to be said that the difference here may not be very great. Yet another reason for creating a classification is for the purpose of making identifications. This occurs in practical situations such as pest or weed control, and for commercial reasons with crop varieties. In this case the characters will be chosen for their ease of use and reliability and for the fact that they provide distinctions between organisms. Hence the character set chosen will have a different orientation and a different classification will result. Just four different purposes for a classification have been discussed, and each produces different groupings. Many authors have claimed that one particular kind of classification can be made which will ideally satisfy all purposes, but this cannot be true. A classification can only be ideal for the purpose for which it is intended. It is necessary to decide in advance what kind of relationship is to be represented, and what the purpose of the classification is, and then to build it accordingly.

Although phenetic classification methods can perfectly well be used to create multi-level hierarchies, they are often used just to create groups at the same level, as for example, when defining the species which belong to a genus. Phylogenetic methods on the other hand attempt to map out a network of relationships, or even to derive an ancestral tree of taxa, complete with a plan of how and where characters changed in the process. Given that the initial data is much the same, the latter is considerably more ambitious.

At the start of a taxonomic project, a list of characters to be considered has to be prepared. Published accounts of the same and related organisms should be studied in order to see what characters were used by other authors in the past. It is equally important to study actual organisms, both in the living state and from preserved specimens in collections. The views of experts about which characters should and should not be considered must be reviewed critically. It may be possible to obtain new character data by using modern techniques, such as electron microscopy, or biochemical methods. It is important to remark that characters are supposed to be *homologous*. This term has various definitions, but the basic idea is that when comparing the characters of different organisms, one must be certain to compare like with like. For closely related organisms, this may not present very much obvious difficulty, and in a great many studies, homology of characters is simply assumed without any attempt at justification. Homology can be argued on the grounds of patterns of development. As an example, the so-called pappus hairs which occur in many species of the Compositae (daisy family) are thought to be the equivalent of the sepals or calyx of other flowering plants (Lawrence, 1951). This family has compound flower heads composed of individual flower heads (florets), and there is often a row of leaf-like 'phyllaries' about the base of the head in the position where sepals would be, but these are not equivalent to sepals.

The selection of characters is a matter which has given rise to much dispute. In phenetic classification, it is often argued that as many characters as possible ought to be used. It is well known that classifications based upon character sets selected from particular parts of organisms, or particular stages on the life cycle, will not necessarily correspond, presumably because different parts of the genome affect different suites of characters, and at different times. This is one argument for using as many characters as possible. It is also hoped that as more characters are employed, the stability will be greater, as discussed earlier. Even apart from considerations of classification, it is a sound principle to include a wide range of characters in a study, simply because characters will be needed for purposes other than classification, such as for descriptions, and for use in identification. In cladistic classifications (p. 68) it is argued that only characters which bear evolutionary significance must be used, and other characters must be ignored. This then raises the problem of how to select such characters.

The question as to whether or not characters should be *weighted* has long been controversial. In cladistic classifications, omission of what are regarded as irrelevant characters is an extreme form of weighting. In any kind of study, there are some kinds of characters which ought to be left out. Meaningless characters must be omitted, such as the time of day that a specimen is collected. There are characters whose variation is so great that they have no meaning, e.g. 'the number of leaves on a tree'. Sets of characters may be found which are strongly correlated with one another merely because they are logically connected; in other words, essentially the same property is being measured in more than one way. For example, there might be a character 'presence of petals' with states 'absent' and 'present' and another for 'number of petals' with states 'none' and '1 or more'. In this rather trivial example, it is clear that the same character is being included twice, and that one version of it ought to be removed, in order to avoid bias. Closely correlated character sets also occur in what are called character complexes. This might be because they all contribute to the same biological function, such as the insect-attracting mechanisms of a flower. Such complexes may be detected by using techniques of character analysis (p. 51). It is possible to argue that such complexes ought to be replaced by one or only a few characters in order to remove bias which might be introduced by effectively using the same character several times over. Nevertheless, in actual taxonomic practice, strongly and genuinely correlated character sets are believed to be of great importance in establishing classifications (Davis and Heywood, 1963). A detailed example of the character complexes which underlie the subfamily classification of the plant family Leguminosae is given in Abbott *et al.* (1985, Chapter 6). In cladistic classification, correlated character sets (synapomorphies, p. 71) are also considered to be important. It is therefore not recommended that correlated characters should be simplified. Equal *a priori* character weighting for phenetic classification is strongly recommended by authors such as Gilmour(1937) and Sneath and Sokal(1973), in the absence of any objective method for weighting characters unequally. In fact, Davies (1981) has shown that characters with initially equal weighting contribute unequally to a phenetic classification according to their inherent information content. Davies calculated the information statistic for the different characters in his study and found that a classification based only on highly informative characters was very little different from a classification derived from the complete character set. In other words, the characters are inherently self-weighting. Once a classification has been formed, then *a postiori* character weighting can be derived from the actual distribution of character states within the different groups. This can be used for various purposes, such as in interactive or matching methods of identification (p. 141).

A problem which affects any classification method, phenetic or phylogenetic, is that of *characterisation*. Even when a character has been chosen, and whether it is weighted or not, the manner in which it is described will substantially affect the resulting classification. Bisby and Nicholls (1977) considered six data sets for the Genisteae (Leguminosae), all based on the same characters, but expressed in different ways which seemed to be of minor importance, and obtained major differences in the classifications. They used the phenetic single link method (see p. 56). These differences were sufficient to account for the discrepancies between seven rival published accounts of the group. As an example from this study, consider a character for the arrangement of branches:

> Branches always opposite, as opposed to
> At least some alternate.

Here are two more ways of expressing the same character:

> At least some branches opposite, with
> Branches always alternate.

And again:

> Branches always opposite
> Some branches alternate and some opposite
> Branches always alternate.

Evidently these three different formulations each stress opposite and alternate branching to different degrees. Other examples are easily constructed. Bias may be introduced by deliberately designing characters in order to emphasise unusual situations. This is not to say that this is inherently bad practice. Subjective choices at this stage of any classification method are hard to avoid, and the only advice which can be offered is to be consistent, and to state explicitly any guidelines that have been followed.

3.2 Phenetic classification

Numerical or mathematical taxonomy began to develop in the 1960s, and has now stabilised into a group of standard mathematical techniques. Most of its applications are, and always were, in industry and commerce rather than in biological taxonomy. Of the available textbooks, Gordon (1981) and Dunn and Everitt (1982) give the mathematical detail, but do not discuss biological applications in any detail. The classic textbook for biological numerical taxonomy is Sneath and Sokal (1973) which contains a full account of the mathematical, philosophical and biological arguments. Abbott *et al.* (1985) provide a good modern biological account with a firm mathematical background. Anderberg (1973), unlike the other texts, gives the complete FORTRAN code of his clustering programs. Romesberg (1984) gives a very complete account of the mathematics and the practical details of clustering, but his text is aimed at scientific research workers in general, and is not specifically intended for biologists.

3.2.1 Character analysis

The techniques described here for investigating the information content in and between characters are an optional preliminary to the formation of classifications. They may give useful insight into the correlations between characters.

If the available characters are mainly or entirely real variables, then a standard statistical measure of correlation, the correlation coefficient (formula, p. 143), may be calculated. Principal components analysis (see p. 61) can also be used to investigate the dependence of quantitative characters. Since taxonomic data is commonly qualitative rather than quantitative, another measure is needed which can be applied to qualitative data. This can be done using the information statistic (Appendix, p. 191). The method for doing this was first published by Estabrook (1967), who described a program called CHARANAL.

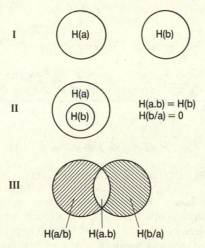

Fig. 3.1   Information held in characters.

The formula given on p. 52 is used for calculating the information content of each character. The information content of characters is represented pictorially in the diagrams of Fig. 3.1. Each complete and separate character is represented by a circle, which may or may not overlap with others. Let the information contained by character *a* be written *H(a)*. In diagram I the two characters do not overlap at all, and the circles are separate. These two characters are entirely independent of each other. In diagram II, character *b* is completely contained in character *a*, so that *a* contains information that is not in *b*, but *b* just duplicates what is in *a*. The general situation is shown in diagram III, where the characters partly overlap. The *conditional information* of character *a* on character *b* is the information held exclusively by *a* when all the information held by *b* is removed, and is written *H(a/b)*. Similarly, the information held by *a* without the contribution of *b* is *H(b/a)*. Finally, the information held by both *a* and *b* is expressed as *H(a.b)*. The areas for *H(a/b)*, *H(a.b)* and *H(b/a)* are shown from left to right in diagram III.

The amount of information held by *a* but not by *b* is found by the usual formula but with character *b* held constant, in state 1, say. Then

$$H(a/b_1) = - \sum_{\substack{\text{all} \\ \text{states} \\ \text{in } a}} p(a/b_1) \log p(a/b_1)$$

This quantity is then summed over all the states of *b* so that

$$H(a/b) = \sum_{\substack{i \\ \text{all} \\ \text{states} \\ \text{in } b}} H(a/b_i) \, p(b_i)$$

with a similar definition for *H(b/a)*. *H(a.b)* is then defined just by subtraction so that

$$H(a.b) = H(a) - H(a/b) = H(b) - H(b/a)$$

The proportion *S* of information shared by two characters as opposed to the total information they hold can be seen in diagram III as the ratio of the unshaded area to the total area

$$S = \frac{H(a.b)}{H(a.b) + H(a/b) + H(b/a)} = \frac{H(a) - H(a/b)}{H(b) + H(a/b)}$$

This value *S* may be regarded as a measure of correlation or similarity between two characters. In order to calculate the information values for actual data sets, allowance has to be made for missing, inapplicable and variable characters. Quantitative characters have to be converted into (pseudo)qualitative characters by dividing them up into ranges (see p. 115).

Table 3.1 summarises some results for the genus *Epilobium*, based on the matrix of Fig. 1.1 and using CHANAL, one of the PANKEY programs. Also shown, for comparison, are separation coefficients (see p. 191). Although neither of the two measures has been normalised to allow for the fact that the characters do not all have the same number of states, they both indicate that character 13 (diameter of flower) is the most informative. This is a quantitative character which has been split into ranges, and different results would be obtained if different ranges were used. Character 14 (flower colour) has the next best information score. In general, the higher scores correspond to characters which are fully scored, have well distributed states and which do not vary within species, as can be seen in the data matrix. In the character pair summary, the highest value for *S* is 1.0 for characters 6 and 12, which is because they have an identical distribution of states i.e. they are exactly correlated. By analogy with the representation of information by circles in Fig. 3.1, 6 and 12 would appear as two circles drawn on top of one another. In cladistic analysis (p. 71) this correlation might be recognised as a synapomorphy. Character pair 4 with 10 shows an *S* value of nearly

Table 3.1 Information in *Epilobium* characters

Character number	Information statistic	Separation coefficient
1	0.9913	0.4102
2	0.8404	0.2051
3	0.7827	0.2308
4	0.8905	0.4615
5	0.8905	0.4615
6	0.3913	0.1538
7	0.9957	0.3846
8	0.3913	0.1538
9	0.8905	0.4615
10	0.9957	0.5385
11	0.7794	0.3846
12	0.3913	0.1538
13	1.4605	0.7692
14	1.1401	0.5000
15	0.8905	0.4615
16	0.9957	0.5385
17	0.9613	0.5128
18	0.7794	0.4102

Character pair summary

a	b	H(a)	H(b)	H(a/b)	H(b/a)	H(a.b)	S
1	2	0.9913	0.8404	0.6200	0.4691	0.3713	0.2542
1	3	0.9913	0.7827	0.4118	0.6563	0.5795	0.4852
1	6	0.9913	0.3913	0.6000	0.0000	0.3913	0.3947
1	12	0.9913	0.3913	0.6000	0.0000	0.3913	0.3947
4	10	0.8905	0.9957	0.8886	0.9938	0.0019	0.0010
4	17	0.8905	0.9613	0.2777	0.3484	0.6128	0.4947
6	12	0.3913	0.3913	0.0000	0.0000	0.3913	1.0000

zero, which almost corresponds with diagram I of Fig. 3.1, since these two characters are almost independent of each other. In the data matrix of Fig. 1.1, it will be seen that in most cases, either one of these characters, but not both, will distinguish a given pair of taxa. Character pairs 1 with 6 and 1 with 12 show an S value of zero for $H(b/a)$, which is the situation of diagram II of Fig. 3.1. This is because the information in character 6 and character 12 is already included in character 1, as can be seen by comparing the rows of the matrix. Not all the results have been shown in the table, but pairs 1 with 3 and 4 with 17 have high values of S. These correlations might be stated in words by saying that species with erect habit tend to have hairy stems, and that if there are glandular hairs on the stem, they tend to occur on the calyx as well. This simple but uncontrived example shows clearly the value of the information statistic for character analysis.

3.2.2 Similarity measures

Before clustering methods can be applied, it is necessary to compute a measure of similarity between two objects. For qualitative characters, the simple *similarity coefficient S* between two objects is defined as the ratio

$$\frac{\text{no. of characters which agree}}{\text{total number of characters}}$$

The value of S is zero when two objects are entirely different, and unity when they are identical. The *dissimilarity coefficient D* is the opposite of this, namely

$$\frac{\text{no. of characters which disagree}}{\text{total number of characters}}$$

The total number of characters means the total number which are known in common between two objects, since they may not show the same set of characters. Characters with missing or inapplicable states are left out. The value of D is unity when two objects are totally different, and zero when they are identical. D may be thought of as an analogy to the distance between two objects. Evidently, $D = 1-S$, and $S = 1-D$.

It may happen that some characters have a negative and positive sense, or describe the presence or absence of something. In which case, if two characters which are being compared both have a negative state, this may not always be considered to be a match. For example, in comparing vegetation samples, the presence of a species in two samples is thought significant, whereas absence from both may be seen as meaningless. Species which could never occur in that particular habitat will always be absent from both samples, and those do not count. In some applications, therefore, negative matches may be omitted. The original use of this kind of similarity was in an ecological application by Jaccard. Beware of the fact that the apparent negative condition of a character state may be nothing more than a form of words. As an example, consider the character 'stem surface' with states 'smooth (glabrous)' or 'hairy' as opposed to 'stem hair presence' with states 'absent' or 'present'. The choice between the simple and the Jaccard coefficient is therefore a subjective matter. One possibility is to regard negative matches as significant when considering a set of closely related objects, and as meaningless for distantly related objects.

The coefficients discussed so far only apply to binary characters which are not variable within the objects. Gower (1971) proposed a mixed coefficient which allows for qualitative binary and multi-state and quantitative characters. Binary qualitative characters are compared as already described. Multi-state characters are compared in essentially the same way. The similarity for quantitative characters, provided there is a single measurement for each of two objects 1 and 2 is calculated as

$$1 - \frac{\text{difference between measurements 1 and 2}}{\text{total range of measurements for character}}$$

A multi-state character is the equivalent of several binary characters. A character with 4 states, for example, is the equivalent to two binary characters.

The mixing of binary with multi-state characters effectively undervalues the multi-state characters, and if it is desired to correct this, multi-state characters should be given a weight greater than unity. The logarithm to base 2 of the number of states is the obvious choice. It is misleading to refer to this process as 'weighting', as in fact all that is happening is that a detectable form of bias is being removed. A formula for combining similarities with weights is given on p. 143.

If there is character variation within objects, the Gower coefficient needs to be modified. If a qualitative character varies differently between two objects, then the similarity is neither 0 nor 1. It can be measured for one character between two given objects as

$$\frac{\text{number of states held in common}}{\text{total number of different states}}$$

For example, for a binary character which in one object is absent or present, and present in the other, the similarity would be 1/2. For 'flower colour' which is 'white' or 'pink' in one and 'pink' or 'red' in the other, the similarity is 1/3.

For quantitative characters, each character can vary over a range of values. When comparing two objects in this character, there may or may not be some overlap in the range of their states. If there is, then the similarity is

$$\frac{\text{overlap between the two ranges}}{\text{overall range between the two objects}}$$

For example, if the leaves in one plant vary from 10 to 18 cm, and in another from 16 to 30, then the overlap is 2 (18-16), the overall range is 20 (30-10) and the similarity is 0.1.

Most of the classification problems in biology involve at least some qualitative characters, but if not, there is a special case. If the characters are all quantitative real variables and without a range of variation, then their values could be treated as if they were points in a multidimensional space, with as many axes as there are characters (N, say). An object could then be represented as a point in this space, and the difference between two objects as the distance between two points, calculated using Pythagoras' theorem for N dimensions. If object i is represented by a point at $(X_{i1}, X_{i2}, \ldots X_{iN})$, the squared distance between objects i and j is

$$(X_{i1}-X_{j1})^2 + \ldots (X_{iN}-X_{jN})^2$$

Take the square root to get the distance and scale it to get it in the range 0 to 1. The result can then be used as a dissimilarity coefficient.

Another statistical measure which might be considered is the correlation coefficient (formula p. 143), but this ranges in value from -1 to +1 and does not have the properties of a metric value i.e. it does not behave like a measure of distance. Its use is not recommended.

The kind of similarity coefficient which is chosen is affected by the type of relationship which the classification is intended to represent. Different methods of calculating similarity will give rise to differing results from clustering, and this choice is partly subjective.

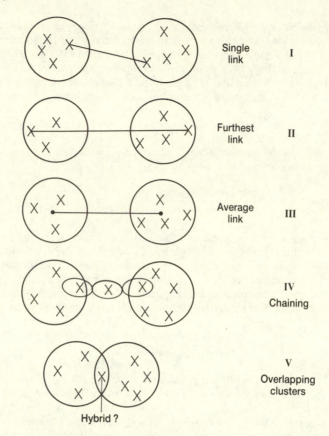

Single link   I

Furthest link   II

Average link   III

IV
Chaining

V
Overlapping clusters

Hybrid ?

Fig. 3.2   Types of agglomerative cluster method.

3.2.3 Clustering methods

There are two main types of clustering method, the *agglomerative* and the *divisive*. These differ according to whether the clusters are arrived at by starting with individual objects and joining them into successively larger groups, or by starting with all objects in one group, and dividing this group into smaller groups. Divisive methods will be considered later (p. 64).

In an agglomerative clustering method, every object is initially in its own group, i.e. the number of groups is the same as the number of objects. The first step is to find the two objects which most resemble one another i.e., the pair which have the highest similarity (or lowest dissimilarity). These two objects are then placed into a group. Subsequent steps involve searching for the next most similar objects, or groups, and combining them, until there is just one group left, which is the group of all objects. Methods differ in the way in which the similarity of two groups is computed. There are several possibilities, illustrated in Fig. 3.2.

The *single link* (or nearest neighbour) method estimates the similarity between two groups by taking the similarity between the two most similar objects, as in diagram I. The opposite extreme is the *complete link* (or furthest neighbour) method, shown in diagram II, where the two most dissimilar objects are selected instead. What may seem intuitively a more reasonable approach is the *average link* method, seen in diagram III, where the average of all the similarities between pairs of objects, one from each group, is computed. The average link method can be modified by weighting the calculation of the similarity of two groups according to the size of the groups. There is also the *centroid* method, which averages the members of each group to find a group centre point, and then takes the similarity between the group centres. All these methods can be seen as variations of a more general method, according to a formula which gives the similarity between two groups in terms of four parameters (Lance and Williams, 1967).

A rather different type of clustering method is based upon the minimisation of sums of squares. If each cluster is viewed as a group of points in two dimensions, as in the diagrams of Fig.3.2, then the 'tightness' of each group can be estimated by finding a centre point for each group and calculating the sum of squares of distances from the centre to each group member. If these sums are added for all groups, then the total should be smaller when the groups are more densely clustered. Hence, the decision on which pair of groups to combine during the cluster building process is based on finding the smallest resulting increase in the sum of squares. The method was first published by Ward(1963). It differs from the other methods in that it provides an estimate of the overall quality of the clustering. Programs (iterative relocation algorithms, e.g. Wishart, 1987) can be written to try and find a global optimum for all possible groupings. This may be done by systematically moving objects from one group to another in the hope of finding a better solution. The difficulty is that the number of possible ways in which groups can be chosen grows astronomically with the number of objects, and that although locally optimal arrangements may be found, these are not related in any way to global solutions. In other words, the only sure way to find the best solution is to search all cases, and this is often impractical. This might possibly be an NP-complete problem (see p. 82).

The tree of classification which results from a clustering is often represented in a dendrogram (also called a phenogram). The dendrograms shown here have the objects (taxa) plotted on one axis and the level of similarity on the other. The nodes of the tree are drawn as vertical lines, and represent the levels at which the corresponding objects or groups of objects are merged. Dendrograms for the *Epilobium* data using the single, complete, and average linkage methods are shown in Figs. 3.3, 3.4 and 3.5. These were prepared using the NTSYS package (Rohlf, 1988). They differ in detail, but have a number of features in common. In general, single linkage tends to exaggerate the similarity between groups and hence may suggest some groups which are unrealistic. Single linkage has a tendency to *chaining*, by which is meant that it forms groups by linking a series of similar objects, as in Fig. 3.2, diagram IV. The resulting cluster is not, geometrically speaking, a coherent group of objects in space, but a more or less linear chain. The corresponding dendrogram will look like a staircase as single objects are split off one at a time from a larger group. Fig. 4.3(b), which is not in fact a dendrogram, shows the kind of pattern which results. By contrast, complete linkage is a conservative method in the sense that it will show the more cohesive clusters but may miss

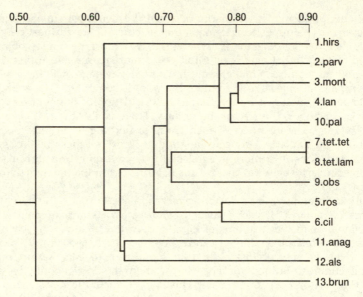

Fig. 3.3   Dendrogram for *Epilobium* using single linkage.

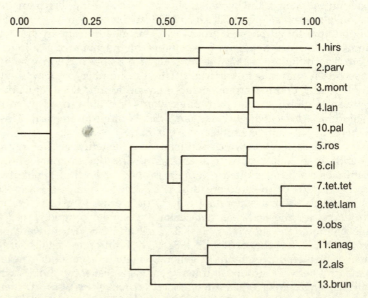

Fig. 3.4   Dendrogram for *Epilobium* using complete linkage.

others which are less clearly defined. Average linkage, not surprisingly, is the compromise between the two extremes and is perhaps used more often than the others. The centroid method suffers from the occurrence of *reversals*, by which is meant that when two groups are combined during the clustering process, it can happen that the level of similarity at which the combination

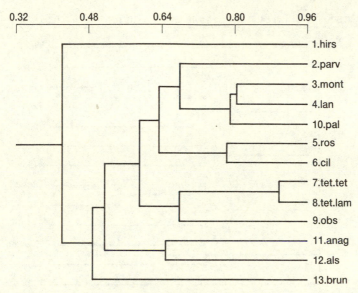

Fig. 3.5   Dendrogram for *Epilobium* using average linkage.

takes place is higher than previously, instead of being always lower, as in other methods. In any of the agglomerative methods, when deciding which groups (or objects) to combine at any stage, it is possible that there is more than one pair of groups with the same similarity score. Most published programs ignore this situation, but in NTSYS and in the SYN-TAX III package (Podani, 1988) the user is given a choice as to what action to take.

No clear recommendation can be given as to which clustering method should be chosen. The fact that a taxonomist will have to choose a particular clustering method and that these produce differing results introduces a subjective element into a phenetic classification. Some authors prefer single linkage, e.g. Abbott *et al.* (1985), and mathematical arguments exist in support of this (Jardine and Sibson, 1971). On the other hand, Dunn and Everitt (1982) remark that average linkage or Ward's method appear to perform best in practice. These methods also have the theoretical advantage that they maximise predictivity (Sneath and Hansell, 1985). The clustering algorithms (except those for relocation) are well behaved as far as computation is concerned. The time taken to process data is generally proportional to the square or the cube of the number of objects, which means that the size of the problem presents no practical difficulty, except perhaps in the labour required to collect the data.

There is obviously a need for an objective method of comparing the results of different cluster methods. One way of doing this is to calculate the *cophenetic correlation coefficient* (Sokal and Rohlf, 1962). This makes use of the *cophenetic matrix*. This is a matrix of the cophenetic similarity between objects. Given a dendrogram, the cophenetic similarity is the similarity level of the common node between two objects. This is often a lower similarity than the direct similarity between two objects, and the dendrogram inevitably tends to distort the true relation between individual pairs of objects. The higher the correlation,

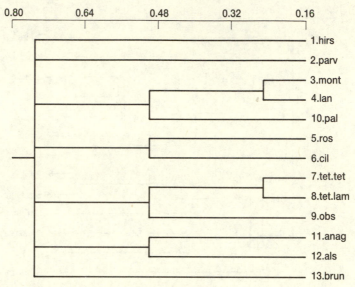

Fig. 3.6   *Epilobium* dendrograms combined in a strict consensus tree.

the less the distortion, and presumably the better the classification. There is no satisfactory statistical test for significance of the correlation, but a value of 0.8 or more is usually considered acceptable. The average linkage method is known to give higher values of correlation than the other methods, and this is borne out by the *Epilobium* examples. The correlation values for single, complete and average linkage were 0.659, 0.652 and 0.767 respectively, for the dendrograms in Figs. 3.3, 3.4 and 3.5. The NTSYS package (Rohlf, 1988) was used to obtain these results.

Various techniques exist for comparing and combining different classifications, and these are known as *consensus* methods (Adams, 1972; Mickevich, 1978; Rohlf, 1982). The algorithms will not be discussed here. An example is shown in Fig. 3.6, which is a *strict consensus* tree of the three dendrograms of Figs. 3.3 to 3.5, produced by NTSYS. This should not be regarded as anything more than a summary of the features of the other three classifications. It should not be supposed that the consensus has somehow plucked a 'correct' classification from among the conflicting results of the three preceding methods. For comments on the statistical significance of consensus trees, see p. 77.

3.2.4 Other methods

3.2.4.1 Ordination methods

A valid criticism of clustering methods is that they set out by assuming that clusters are present. There are alternative geometrical methods, also known as *ordination* or *multi-dimensional scaling* methods, which avoid this assumption. Suppose that the n characters of the objects to be classified can be represented as variables in an n-dimensional space. Each character could be plotted along a separate axis and then clusters would be visible as groups of points in space. This presents no difficulty if the characters are all quantitative numeric, and provided that no more than three are involved. Of course, for more than three variables, it is impractical to plot the objects in space. By using *principal components analysis* it is possible, however, to transform the variables so that, in many cases, much of the total variation is concentrated in the first few dimensions. At the same time, the transformation removes correlation between the old variables and produces new ones which are independent.

Suppose that the initial variables are x_1, x_2 up to x_n. Transform these into new variables y_1 to y_n by a linear transformation with suitable multipliers a_{ij} such that

$$y_1 = a_{11}x_1 + a_{12}x_2\ldots + a_{1n}x_n$$

and similarly for y_2 to y_n. In order to be able to calculate the multipliers a, choose them so that the variance in the new variable y is maximised. This also requires that the values of a, regarded as vectors, are normalised and made orthogonal. This is enough to enable the a's to be computed. The mathematical details are given in Gordon(1981) or Dunn and Everitt (1982). The computation involves finding of eigenvectors (the new variables y) and eigenvalues of a symmetrical matrix. The eigenvalues λ_1 to λ_n come out in descending order of size, and are proportional to the variance contained in each of the new variables y, so that it is easy to see how much variation has been summarised in each y. In the most favourable situation it can happen that some 80% or more of the total variation is contained in the first three variables, so that two-dimensional plots of y_1 against y_2, and similarly y_2 against y_3 and y_1 against y_3 will allow visual inspection of the points for clusters. The problem with this method as it stands is that it requires strictly quantitative characters, and is therefore inapplicable to most taxonomic classification problems.

Fortunately, there is an alternative formulation known as *principal coordinate analysis*, which can be applied to mixed characters. For an explanation of the mathematics, see Gower (1966). Briefly however, the starting point is a matrix of dissimilarities between objects. Each dissimilarity element d_{ij} in the matrix is replaced by $-0.5d_{ij}{}^2$. The matrix is then 'double centred' which means that the row and column means are subtracted from each element and the grand mean is added on. Programs to do this are available in numerical taxonomy packages such as NTSYS. The rest of the analysis then proceeds as before. The *Epilobium* data was used to compute principal coordinates using NTSYS and Figs. 3.7 and 3.8 show plots of the new variables 1 against 2 and 2 against 3, respectively. The transformed variables (eigenvectors) are shown in Table 3.2. The accumulated percentage variation in the first three vectors in this example is only 53%, so this means that the plots in Figs. 3.7 and 3.8 present only about half the character data. Even if the analysis had performed better than this, the plots would still need to be interpreted with caution since the method will sometimes misrepresent taxonomic distance. In other words, closer relationships may not always be represented by shorter distances, and more distant relationships by greater distances, and the actual distances between points on the plots may be unreliable. In spite of these reservations, the principal coordinate plots do reflect some of the same features which were seen in the clusters found previously, such as the association of species 3,4 and 10.

If the distortion of taxonomic distance in principal coordinates is

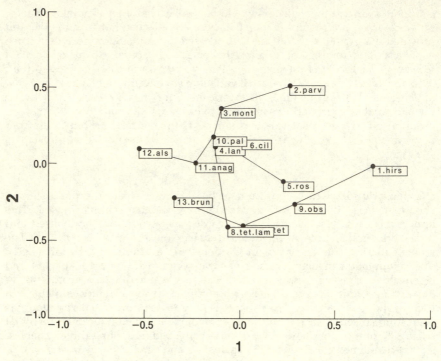

Fig. 3.7   Principal coordinates 1 & 2 for *Epilobium*.

unacceptable, there is an alternative method known as *non-metric multi-dimensional scaling* (Kruskal, 1964 a and b). In this case the scaled taxonomic distances in the resulting plots are monotonic with respect to the dissimilarity matrix. This is to say that greater or lesser taxonomic distances between objects will be preserved and scaled with greater or lesser distances on the plot. In this method it is not variance which is estimated but a heuristic function of the difference between actual and transformed distances, known as *stress*. The algorithm is of an iterative type, which starts by trying to fit a random set of distances, computes a correction, and then converges quite rapidly on a solution. According to Rohlf (1988) the results are generally rather similar to those of principal coordinates analysis.

Correspondence analysis (see Greenacre, 1984) is another form of ordination method which can be used to group both objects by their characters and characters by objects. This approach is appropriate to ecological problems such as vegetation analysis, e.g. Hill *et al.* (1975), but can also be applied to taxonomy. A botanical example is described by Guittoneau and Roux (1978) and a palaeontological example by Gaspard and Mullon (1980).

3.2.4.2 Minimum spanning trees
There is another geometrical way of looking for clusters, known as the *minimum spanning tree*. In mathematical terms, this is simply a graph which connects each object with the next most similar object. This is

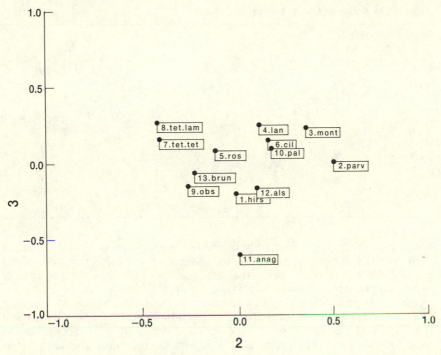

Fig. 3.8 Principal coordinates 2 & 3 for *Epilobium*.

Table 3.2 Principal coordinates for *Epilobium*

First 3 eigenvectors

1	0.7026	−0.0092	−0.2121
2	0.2657	0.5093	−0.0003
3	−0.0959	0.3617	0.2253
4	−0.1289	0.1136	0.2453
5	0.2316	−0.1140	0.0781
6	0.0157	0.1579	0.1433
7	0.0201	−0.4028	0.1595
8	−0.0606	−0.4144	0.2702
9	0.2872	−0.2556	−0.1552
10	−0.1364	0.1747	0.0918
11	−0.2280	0.0052	−0.6065
12	−0.5289	0.0951	−0.1711
13	−0.3441	−0.2215	−0.0683

Eigenvalues

Number	Percent variation	Accumulated percent variation
1	22.5	22.5
2	17.4	39.9
3	13.4	53.3

Table 3.3 Minimum spanning tree for *Epilobium*

Objects (species) connected		Distance (dissimilarity)
1.hirs	9.obs	0.6199
9.obs	7.tet.tet	0.7111
7.tet.tet	8.tet.lam	0.8957
8.tet.lam	4.lan	0.7056
4.lan	3.mont	0.8013
4.lan	10.pal	0.7913
3.mont	2.parv	0.7764
4.lan	6.cil	0.6870
6.cil	5.ros	0.7795
10.pal	11.anag	0.6421
11.anag	12.als	0.6468
7.tet.tet	13.brun	0.5261

easily computed, beginning with the object pair which is closest i.e. least dissimilar. These two objects are then considered to be joined by an edge of the graph. The next object to join is that which is closest to any of those already in the graph, but in such a way as no two points already in the graph are joined again, so that the graph cannot contain loops. The minimum spanning tree for the *Epilobium* similarity matrix is given in Table 3.3. It can be seen that the dissimilarity is not always greater from one step to the next, because of the need to avoid loops. A convenient way to plot the minimum spanning tree is to superimpose it on a principal coordinate plot, as has been done in Fig. 3.7. Any groups which are formed by visual inspection of the clusters in this plot would be expected to be closely connected in the minimum spanning tree, as for example with the species 3,4 and 10.

3.2.4.3 Divisive classification methods
Divisive methods have been much used for *association analysis*, i.e. the analysis of quadrats of vegetation in ecology or phytosociology. Divisive methods differ from agglomerative methods (p. 56) in that they start by considering all objects as belonging to one group, and then proceed by successively dividing this group into smaller groups. Some criterion is needed for deciding which division is the best to choose. This is not generally based on similarity coefficients, and a variety of different measures could or have been used (see CLUSTAN or SYN-TAX III). Possible measures include:

    1) Minimum sum of squares, as in Ward's method (p. 57).

    2) Measures used in association analysis, such as the χ^2 statistic (Williams and Lambert, 1959), or a measure based on the information statistic (Lance and Williams, 1968).

    3) Separation coefficients, or maximum predictivity (see below).

Unlike agglomerative methods, with divisive methods it is customary to provide a stopping rule. That is to say, instead of continuing the division process until every object is left in a group of size one, a decision is made to cut off the process at an earlier stage. This might be because the number of possible groups grows exponentially with each division, and it is impractical to explore them all; or because only the major groupings are actually wanted.

The rule might be chosen to limit the number of groups, or to limit the number of hierarchical levels, or by some cut-off value of the division criterion. It may also be considered necessary to carry out a relocation procedure (p. 57) on the hierarchy after the division process is complete, since this may enable better solutions to be found.

Many divisive methods have been deliberately constructed so as to produce monothetic classifications. This is done by selecting groups according to the states of one or more characters. For classifications of plants and animals this is not normally done since polythetic groupings are preferred, but it is suitable for some applications, such as in association analysis. In such cases, the characters of the objects are actually the frequencies of occurrence of various species, and it makes sense to choose groupings which correspond to individual species, since the groups will then be easily identified. There is an analogy here to the heuristics used in the construction of identification keys (p. 127). See also Section 5.7 on matching keys.

Since we have already stated that predictivity is an important property of a good classification, then it makes sense to use this as the basis of a method of classification. Gower (1974) used a measure of predictivity as a basis for his method of *maximal predictive classification*. Sneath and Hansell (1985) show mathematically that the highest value of Gower's predictivity is obtained by using an unweighted average link clustering method, or if weighted, to a sum of squares clustering.

Suppose that n objects with m characters are divided into k clusters. If we consider only one cluster and examine the objects within it, we can survey the states of characters to find which occur the most frequently. With these states we can define a *predictor*, which is an object (normally fictitious) which possesses the commonest states of the characters in the cluster. The notion of this predictor taxon rather resembles the traditional idea of the idealised 'type' taxon. Using this predictor, the real objects in the cluster can be compared with it, and the number of characters which agree can be counted. This is the number of correct predictions in the cluster, and is also the same as the sum of the similarities between the predictor and all the members of the group, multiplied by m, the number of characters. Summing this quantity over all clusters, we obtain a value W_k, which is positive and has a maximum possible value of nm. This is the total number of correct predictions for k clusters. This measure represents the total agreement within the clusters, but is not by itself adequate for choosing the best classification of k clusters since it increases with k.

W_k needs to be balanced by some measure of the disagreement between clusters. Consider the objects in cluster k and add up the number of correct predictions from the other $(k-1)$ clusters. Sum this for k clusters, to obtain a quantity which is denoted B_k. Evidently we want W_k to be high and B_k to be low, so calculate W_k-B_k. There is a further correction needed, in order to correct for homogeneity. If the k clusters each contained objects which were identical to one another, W_k-B_k would still not be zero (Gower, 1973). The final criterion for maximum predictivity is:

$$W_k - B_k - n\log_2 k[1 - (k-2)/2k(k-1)]$$

Gower described what he called a transfer algorithm for maximising the criterion. The idea is simply to try and improve the best known value for k clusters by shifting some object from out of one cluster into another, as in the iterative relocation algorithms mentioned above (p. 57). Different maxima are found by starting from different trial clusters, and so Gower suggests three ways of starting:

1) With groups chosen by the user.
2) By random groupings.
3) By computation.

Start with the two most similar objects, and put each one into separate groups to form two groups. One object can be put into each remaining cluster by picking in turn objects which have the greatest average difference from objects already chosen. Any remaining objects are then put into whichever group they most resemble.

No algorithm is known for reliably finding the optimum except by searching all cases. This becomes rapidly impractical with larger values of n, even at the speed of modern computers. There does not seem to be a published proof, but this looks likely to be an NP-complete problem (p. 82). This is to say that the computational problems are severe and probably insuperable.

Table 3.4   Maximal predictive classification of *Epilobium*

No. of groups	Value of criterion	Group membership
2	43.50	(1 9) (2 3 4 5 6 7 8 10 11 12 13)
3	36.06	(1 2 9) (3 4 7 8 12) (5 6 10 11 13)
4	40.46	(1) (2 3 6) (4 7 8 9 12) (5 10 11 13)
5	41.50	(1 5 9) (2 3 4 6 12) (7 8) (10 11) (13)
6	53.62	(1) (2 3 4 10) (5 6) (7 8 9) (11 12) (13)
7	56.46	(1) (2 3 4 10) (5 6) (7 8 9) (11) (12) (13)
8	57.18	(1) (2) (3 4 10) (5 6) (7 8 9) (11) (12) (13)
9	57.03	(1) (2) (3 4 10) (5 6) (7 8) (9) (11) (12) (13)
10	55.08	(1) (2) (3 4 10) (5 6) (7) (8) (9) (11) (12) (13)
11	54.73	(1) (2) (3 4 10) (5) (6) (7) (8) (9) (11) (12) (13)
12	53.89	(1) (2) (3 4) (5) (6) (7) (8) (9) (10) (11) (12) (13)
13	52.83	(1) (2) (3) (4) (5) (6) (7) (8) (9) (10) (11) (12) (13)
CON	53.64	(1) (2) (3 4 10) (5 6) (7 8 9) (11 12) (13)
A(8)	43.46	(1 2 9) (3 4) (5 6) (7 8) (12) (11) (10 13)
B(7)	37.09	(1) (2) (3) (4 10) (5 6 7 8) (9) (11 12 13)
C(7)	30.56	(1 2 7 8) (3 4) (5 6) (9 10) (11 12) (13)

Values of the criterion have been computed for *k*=2 to 13 for the *Epilobium* matrix and the results are shown in Table 3.4. The entry shown is maximised separately for each value of *k*, and the best is for *k*=8. Not surprisingly this is almost identical with the arrangement for the consensus of clustering on the same data (Fig. 3.6) which is shown lower in the table, against the label CON. As expected, because average link clustering is known to maximise predictivity, it is also very close to the groups found for average linking (Fig. 3.5).

Applications of this method have been surprisingly few, considering how often stress has been laid on the importance of predictivity. There are studies of the classification of yeasts by Barnett, Bascomb and Gower (1975) and of the Epacridaceae by Correll (1977). It may be possible, as suggested by Gower, to extend the method to cover hierarchies instead of just simple clusters. The criterion of maximum predictivity might also be used in cladistic analysis to help decide between cladograms of equal parsimony (p. 77).

3.2.4.4 Non-hierarchical classification
In the previous discussion (p. 4) it was argued that although non-hierarchical classifications occur in everyday language, they are not appropriate in taxonomy. To speak of non-hierarchical classification is perhaps misleading; what is of interest is overlapping or partially hierarchical classifications. There is one situation where this is of practical value, which is when hybrids are suspected or known to be present among the objects to be classified. If the parents of a hybrid are in two different clusters, then the clusters might be considered to overlap, with the hybrid as the object which belongs to both clusters, as in Fig. 3.2, diagram V. Jardine and Sibson (1968) invented an algorithm to search for overlapping clusters, which they successfully applied to finding hybrids in the genus *Solanum*. The details will not be given here, but the algorithm asks the user to specify the degree of overlapping (maximum number of objects which can occur in more than one cluster) and a threshold value of similarity which is the minimum for the formation of clusters. In the special case where the degree of overlap is set to zero, the method reduces to the single linkage clustering algorithm. The original method made heavy demands on the computer, but Cole and Wishart (1970) have made an improved version. In the KDEND program in the CLUSTAN package (Wishart, 1987) up to 60 objects are allowed.

3.2.5 Available program packages

Readers should beware that the comments made in this section may become out of date rapidly, as new versions of software packages are produced. One author on clustering methods (Anderberg, 1973) has actually published the FORTRAN code for his programs. This is not as helpful as it seems, since some of the programs have uncorrected errors in them. Apart from this, three major packages, CLUSTAN, NTSYS and SYN-TAX III, were available for review at the time of writing. All three were tested on IBM-compatible microcomputer versions, but all exist in versions for minicomputers or mainframes as well. All three can be run in either interactive or batch modes. In each case, the main emphasis is on agglomerative methods and ordination, rather than divisive methods, and in each case, the programs can accept either raw data or a (dis)similarity matrix from an external file.

CLUSTAN (version 3.3, Wishart, 1987) is the most comprehensive of the three, and has the widest range of different algorithms. It gives the impression of being aimed at industrial and commercial uses rather than for taxonomists. It employs a special command language of its own. The interaction is by simple scrolling of output on the screen, and the commands are not intrinsically difficult to learn, but nevertheless the user interface is, by modern standards, not particularly friendly. Similarity or dissimilarity coefficients can be computed by CLUSTAN or read from external files, but there is not a great deal of provision for the mixed character types which are needed for much of biological taxonomy. The effect of this has been that a number of potentially useful programs could not be applied to the standard *Epilobium* data set since all characters in the input file were required to be real variables. This is the case, for example, with the RELOCATE option for iterative improvement of classifications. The documentation does say that it is planned to remove this restriction. Dendrograms and other diagrams can be output in a line printer mode or to a plotter, if available.

SYN-TAX III (Podani, 1988) provides a good range of programs for cluster analysis, ordination and comparison of classifications (consensus methods) and is designed for the use of taxonomists and ecologists. The user interface is again not difficult to use, but shows signs of having been updated from an earlier punched-card system. One feature special to SYN-TAX III is a program for clustering with measures of homogeneity, instead of similarity. As in CLUSTAN, there are several different methods for divisive clustering and a program for relocation of existing partitions. Dendrograms and other diagrams can be output in a line printer mode.

NTSYS (version 1.50, Rohlf, 1988) is again intended for the use of taxonomists, and is better oriented to interactive use on microcomputers than the other packages. It includes a comprehensive range of programs for clustering, ordination and for comparison of trees. The documentation usefully provides a short account of the mathematical background with each program. NTSYS is organised with menus, windows and help screens and uses the full screen in colour, if available. Diagrams and plots can be output to the screen or to a variety of printers in graphics mode. NTSYS was used in preference, for the production of various clustering and ordination examples in this book.

3.3 Phylogenetic and cladistic classifications

Entia non sunt multiplicanda praeter necessitatem. William of Occam (d. 1349)

3.3.1 Introduction

In this section, we consider computer methods which can be used to help construct classifications which involve, in some sense or other, ideas about evolution. It is important to realise that there is no absolute obligation to choose an evolutionary method of classification, as we can equally well choose to construct other kinds of classification (see the discussion above, p. 44). There exist several myths about evolutionary classifications which are repeated in the literature. For example, Mayr (1969) in his classic textbook on taxonomy, states that the 'most important aim of evolutionary classification is . . . to combine maximal information content with maximal ease of retrieval of this information'. These criteria are important aims in any type of classification, but evolutionary classifications are certainly not the only types of classification to have such properties. The quotation continues, 'The evolutionist believes that a classification consistent with our reconstruction of phylogeny has a better chance of meeting these objectives than any other method of classification'. Such beliefs are certainly widespread, but the fact is that each type of classification will perform better at the purposes it is aimed at, and no one classification method exists which can satisfy all the various conflicting criteria at once, even though in practice the differences may be small. Wiley (1981) expresses a similar belief: 'The best general classification of organisms is one that exactly reflects the genealogical relationships among these organisms' (p.1). A similar point of view can be found in botanical literature, e.g. Takhtajan (1980) who says ' . . . it is evolutionary or phylogenetic classification which is really synthetic and acquires all the explanatory, heuristic and predictive value and can therefore serve as the best reference system'. For a contrasting viewpoint, see Chapter 10 in Abbott *et al.* (1985), where classifications based on theories of genealogy are opposed because 1) there is 'no certain method for deducing the phylogenetic history', and 2) 'even were the history known, to include either its branching pattern . . . or its time-scale into the classification would in many cases conflict with the classification's information property of storing the pattern of homogeneities and discontinuities found among the organisms today'. Stace (1989) remarks that cladistic classifications are not necessarily the most predictive. Also, Davis and Heywood (1963) remark that 'a characteristic of post-Darwinian taxonomy has been the construction of phylogenetic trees on extremely dubious evidence'. They prefer a 'natural' system, by which they mean classifications based on overall resemblance.

Mayr, and also other authors, make a distinction between *evolutionary* or *phylogenetic* classifications and those which are *cladistic*. A *cladistic* classification is arranged according to the branching points in the genealogy of the organisms. There is of course, historically, only one such pattern, and it would be of enormous interest if we could, in general, discover precisely and unequivocally what that pattern was. This approach ignores the effect of differing rates of evolution in different lines, and in the assignment of ranks to the branches, equates genealogical distance with genetic distance, which is often not correct. The taxa in one branch of the evolutionary tree may remain more or less unchanged over a long period of time, whereas taxa in another branch from the same common ancestor may have evolved and diversified greatly in the same period. Mayr proposes that this situation should be taken into account in classifications. He uses the term 'evolutionary' to describe this kind of classification, but readers should beware of the different meanings given to the words 'evolutionary' and 'phylogenetic' by various authors in this context. Unfortunately, the methods which produce this kind of classification are largely subjective, and cannot be expressed in algorithms, so there is nothing more that can be said here. On the other hand, parts of the cladistic method can be computerised. The following discussion will not include any dialogue about methods which apply to molecular data, as these are rather specialised. Cladistic classification is normally associated with the name of Hennig (1966), who published some of the main ideas involved, although his text is not recommended as an introduction. It is generally assumed that when a hypothesis has been put forward about the evolution of a group, this will then be used to create a classification. This is not necessarily so, however, and there is a school of so-called 'pattern cladists' who use cladistic methods without claiming that they should be used to create classifications.

There is a general belief among cladists that groups in classifications ought to be monophyletic. Whether the taxonomic groups created in a classification based on a cladogram are monophyletic or not does not affect the procedures for obtaining the cladogram. However, Cronquist (1987) forcefully makes the point that some existing, widely accepted groups are probably paraphyletic and that it is proper that they should be so. One of his examples concerns the Monocotyledons, which are thought to have derived from the Dicotyledons. If so, the Dicotyledons are a paraphyletic group which has been universally accepted for several centuries!

3.3.2 Definitions

A tree diagram in which the vertical scale represents time, the nodes represent species (current or extinct) and a line which joins two nodes represents descent or ancestry, is called a *cladogram*. These are normally drawn with no more than two descendants to each ancestor, but multiway branches are possible. In fact, although cladograms often refer to species, each node could also be a genus, a family, or a taxon at any other rank, provided that all nodes have the same rank. The nodes in a cladogram may represent either living or extinct taxa, and actual or hypothetical (reconstructed) taxa. It is also possible to draw a branching diagram which does not have a root and a direction to it, and this is called a *network*. A network becomes a tree when one of its nodes is chosen as a root. If all organisms in a branching genealogical tree or part of it have the same single common ancestor, and all the descendants of that ancestor are included, then that group of organisms

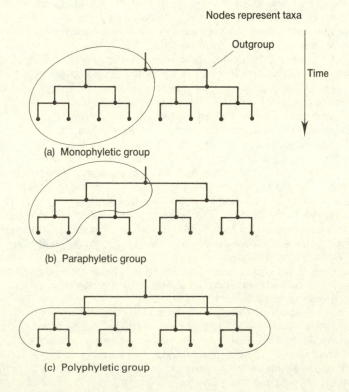

Fig. 3.9 Types of phyletic group.

is said to be *monophyletic*, Fig. 3.9(a). A monophyletic group of taxa is called a *clade*. When a group of organisms all have the same common ancestor, but not all the descendants are included, then the group is *paraphyletic*, Fig. 3.9(b). If a group of organisms includes two or more complete branches from different parts of a tree, but does not include the common ancestor, then the group is said to be *polyphyletic*, Fig. 3.9(c). These definitions are given in terms of the tree structure only. Other definitions have sometimes been given by other authors. The term *character* was defined above (p. 2), but some authors in cladistics use the word 'character' to mean the state of a character. This non-standard usage is confusing and is not recommended. An *outgroup* of a clade is another monophyletic group with the same ancestor as the clade e.g. the species in the group NOT circled in Fig. 3.9(a). A *sister-group* of a clade is the outgroup which is closest genealogically to the clade. If a character varies within the taxa in a clade, the character state which appears in the ancestor is said to be *primitive* or *ancestral*, and the different state(s) which appear in descendants are said to be *advanced* or *derived*. If two taxa both have the same state of a character and this state is primitive, then this is called a *symplesiomorphy* (literally, shared primitive state). Conversely, if two taxa share an advanced (apomorphic) character state, then this is called a *synapomorphy*. One of the contributions of Hennig was to point out the significance of synapomorphy. If two species both show the same advanced character state (synapomorphy), then this is evidence of common ancestry. If two species share a primitive character (symplesiomorphy), this is also evidence of common ancestry. However, if a group of taxa has symplesiomorphic characters this is not sufficient evidence of monophyly because of the possibility that there existed other taxa in the clade which are now extinct. The group defined by the symplesiomorphies might be paraphyletic. When a cladogram has been constructed as a hypothesis of the ancestry of a group, the differences of the states of many characters between one species and its relatives will be expected to correlate with the structure of the tree. It often happens that there are characters whose observed character-state distributions do not fit with the tree, and this situation is called *homoplasy*.

In the Table 3.5, the *Epilobium* data matrix has been coded for a cladistic analysis. This matrix has been chosen because it is the unifying example used throughout this book. Unfortunately, there are no arguments available to help decide whether some characters are significant for evolution and others not; so the complete character set has been used. There is no way of knowing in advance how many characters are necessary as a basis for the construction of a satisfactory cladogram, but it is often difficult to find enough. In this case, 18 characters for 13 taxa is not excessive. There is also no evidence available as to which character states are primitive and which are advanced, so initially states have been arbitrarily coded as 0 for primitive and 1 (and 2) for advanced. On the basis of the apomorphies in the table, we can attempt to construct a tree which fits. As an example, consider just the first three species, A,B and C. First pick out groups of species which have advanced character states. For example, synapomorphies occur which group species AB (characters 3,4 and 17), BC (10) and ABC (12 and 15). There are also the single species A and C which show advanced (apomorphic) states (characters 8,9,13,14 and 16, and character 7, respectively). These can be treated as possible clades containing just one species. The complete list of species groups is then A,C,AB,BC and ABC. Each of these groups ought to be a monophyletic group, or clade. In

Table 3.5   *Epilobium* matrix for cladistics

Primitive state = 1, advanced states = 2(3), ? variable.

Taxon		Characters																	
		1	2	3	4	5	6	7	8	9	10	11	12	13	14	15	16	17	18
0. ANCESTOR	X	1	1	1	1	1	1	1	1	1	1	1	1	1	1	1	1	1	1
1. hirsutum	A	3	2	2	2	1	1	1	2	1	1	1	2	3	3	2	1	2	1
2. parviflorum	B	3	?	2	2	1	1	1	1	1	1	1	2	2	3	2	2	2	1
3. montanum	C	3	?	1	1	1	1	2	1	1	2	1	2	2	2	1	1	1	1
4. lanceolatum	D	3	2	1	1	2	1	2	1	1	1	1	2	2	2	1	1	1	1
5. roseum	E	3	2	1	2	2	1	2	1	1	1	1	2	2	2	1	1	2	1
6. ciliatum	F	3	2	1	2	2	1	2	1	1	1	1	2	1	1	1	2	2	1
7. tetragonum ssp. t	G	3	2	1	1	2	1	1	1	2	2	1	2	1	2	1	2	1	1
8. t. ssp. lamyi	H	3	2	1	1	2	1	2	1	2	1	1	2	2	2	1	2	1	1
9. obscurum	I	3	2	1	1	2	1	?	1	2	2	2	2	3	3	1	2	2	1
10. palustre	J	3	?	?	1	1	1	?	1	1	1	2	2	2	2	1	1	1	1
11. anagallidifolium	K	2	1	?	1	2	1	1	1	1	1	1	2	1	3	1	1	1	2
12. alsinifolium	L	2	1	?	1	2	1	2	1	1	1	2	2	2	2	1	1	1	2
13. brunnescens	M	1	2	1	1	2	2	?	1	1	2	2	1	2	2	1	2	1	2
Apomorphies, groups of species with advanced character states		C … J	A D … I	A B	A B E F	D … I K … M	M	C … F H L	A	A G … I	B C F – L M	G H L	A … L	A H	A I K	A … D	A E C … – M	A B E F – I	K L M

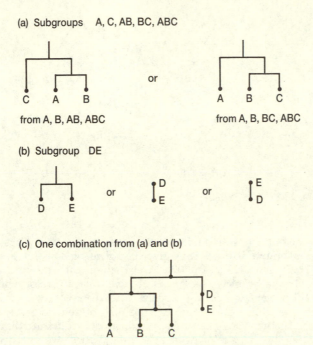

Fig. 3.10 Construction of cladogram from consistent characters.

fact, trees can only be drawn with A,B,AB and ABC (on which BC does not fit) or with A,B,BC and ABC (where AB does not fit) as in Fig. 3.10(a). This is an example of homoplasy. A set of *compatible* characters on which these consistent clades are based, such as the character set 3,4,7-9 and 12-17, is known as a *clique*. Character 10, corresponding to the group BC, has been dropped. Suppose we decide to add the species D and E to the cladogram. We find support for all three possibilities for D and E, as shown in Fig. 3.10(b). A possible cladogram drawn with these 5 characters is seen in Fig. 3.10(c), where it was decided to put D before E. There is in fact no conclusive evidence for this, and E could have been put before D, as they both have the same number of advanced and primitive states, and so the clade DE is said to be *unresolved*, i.e. it is not possible to decide on the exact relation between D and E.

At this point, it is necessary to point out the practical problems which stem from the methods as proposed originally by Hennig (Felsenstein,1984):

1) A method is needed for knowing conclusively which character states are ancestral i.e. to decide character polarity.

2) Some method is needed for handling characters whose states do not exactly fit the proposed tree, i.e. show homoplasy. Such characters will show one or more reversals, i.e. changes from advanced to primitive. Looking at this another way, homoplasy corresponds roughly to what is called convergence and/or parallelism. Various approaches to this are considered below.

To this should be added a third difficulty:

3) In a considerable number of cases, the rooted tree is known not to be

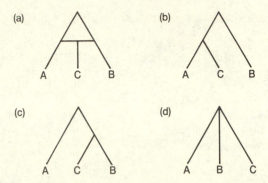

Fig. 3.11   Models for the evolution of hybrids.

an accurate model of how evolution took place. In plants, species frequently have a hybrid origin. Baum (1984) gives a figure of 30% for angiosperms, and Stace (1987) estimates 50 to 70%. A cladogram can still be drawn when hybridisation has taken place, see Fig. 3.11. The true picture of what occurred is represented in diagram a, where species C was derived by crossing species A and B. The horizontal lines represent the flow of genetic material between the branches. The genealogy can be approximated by drawing diagrams with binary forks, as in b and c, or even by having a three-way branch, as in d. The trouble is that the inheritance of characters is no longer monophyletic. In diagram b, characters of species B can recur in the descendants of C, even though these descendants are not in the same clade. The same difficulty still arises if the branching is drawn as in diagram c or d. To put this another way, such characters will not fit on any simple branching cladogram because they are incompatible with any such tree. This is one possible cause of homoplasy. Sneath (1975) discusses the problem of reticulate evolution in more detail.

3.3.3 Choice of a group, characters and polarity

Logically, the first task is to choose a group of species which are monophyletic. How do we know which taxa belong to a clade? The answer is that we can only make a hypothesis, i.e. make a reasonable assumption. It is often argued that a group is monophyletic because all taxa within it have the same derived state in one or more characters, i.e. they all share at least one synapomorphous character. This kind of argument may be plausible, but it is not direct evidence; it is just a credible hypothesis. There may be some direct evidence from breeding, the idea being that the species which interbreed most readily to form hybrids are the most closely related. The relationship here though is genetic rather than genealogical. Unfortunately, cases are known where closely related taxa cannot interbreed, whereas more distantly related taxa can, so this criterion is not reliable (Stace, 1975, p. 10). The most convenient evidence for monophyly is morphological, i.e. members of a clade are taxa which resemble one another, or have phenetic similarity. The problem here is that there may be convergence, i.e. external similarity brought about by environment, which may cover up the genealogical difference. It may well happen that the initial hypothesis about which taxa form a clade will be modified as a result of later steps in the analysis, and that the investigator may need to return and revise this initial decision.

For a cladistic classification, the only characters which can be used are those which reflect evolutionary history. Other characters are irrelevant. How do we know which characters are the right ones? Unfortunately, there is no algorithm for doing this, and the characters must be chosen subjectively by an experienced taxonomist. As a matter of principle, characters must be homologous and in this context, it is important to use a definition which does not already include evolutionary arguments (Wiley, 1981). There are certain kinds of correlated characters which have no evolutionary basis. These have already been discussed (p. 49). Most cladistic algorithms permit characters to be binary or multistate, but not all of them permit characters in which there is variability within a taxon (polymorphism), so polymorphic characters may not be of use. Quantitative characters normally have to be converted and expressed as qualitative characters before they can be used.

The next problem is to decide the *polarity* of the states of the characters, i.e. which character states are primitive and which are advanced. Some cladistic methods are *ordered* methods, and require the polarity of character states to be decided in advance, and others are not (unordered). If suitable fossils were available for study, polarity could be decided without any doubt, but this is practically never the case. There is not usually any absolute ruling as to whether a state is primitive or advanced in general, and the polarity often has to be decided in respect of the group under study. In a different group, the same character could have a different polarity. Standard textbooks on taxonomy often list the standard assumptions that may be made about character polarity, e.g. for plants, in Radford *et al.* (1974, Chapter 27). As an example, for plants it is generally believed that woody stems are more primitive than herbaceous ones. There may be developmental reasons to show which is the primitive state, e.g. at least at some initial stage, simple leaves must have preceded compound ones. However, in Australian species of the genus *Acacia* (leguminous shrubs), it is believed that compound leaves are primitive. Obviously, if the genus began with compound leaves, it must have derived from something with simple leaves at an earlier date, but with respect to that genus, compound is believed to be primitive.

The various lines of argument which may be used to assign character polarities are given below. Unfortunately, none of them is totally reliable, and they are all more or less subjective (Stuessy and Crisci, 1984).

1) Common equals primitive. The idea is that the character state which is commonest among the extant taxa should be the primitive one. As an example, Sporne (1954) surveyed the frequency of character states among dicotyledonous plants. For example, the commonest number of flower petals is 5. Having 5 petals would be primitive as long as there had not been massive extinction of species with other numbers of petals. Since there is no way of knowing whether that has been the case, this criterion is not really valid.

2) Ontogeny. The idea is that as the juvenile forms of animals or plants develop, the sequence of states which their characters show will recapitulate the history of the evolution of the characters. This is plausible in the sense that juvenile characters tend to be more general (primitive) and adult characters more specialised (advanced). If characters change by mutation, however,

this is just as likely to affect any stage of an organism. Mayr (1969) states categorically that polarity cannot be deduced from ontogeny, and Stace (1989) also states that it is unreliable. Andre (1988) gives several examples which contradict the rule and states that there exist many more.

3) Outgroups. Given that a character varies within the supposedly mono-phyletic group under consideration, where it shows both the primitive and the advanced states in different species, and the same character is constant in an outgroup, then the state which occurs in the outgroup is the primitive one. Remembering that an outgroup is being assumed to have a common ancestor with the clade which is being considered, Fig. 3.9, then this argument reduces as follows. If the outgroup has very few species in it compared with the clade, then what is being assumed is that the ancestor of both is rather much like the species in the outgroup, which is very little different from the assumption already made. If the outgroup and the clade are of comparable size, then evidently the 'advanced' state is only found in the clade, and not in the outgroup, which has the 'primitive' character only. This is just criterion 1 again in disguise, i.e. common equals primitive. In other words, this criterion is redundant or unreliable. In spite of this, the outgroup criterion is popular in cladistic studies, and is used in many of the computer programs. It should be regarded as a way of stating the assumptions to be made about which states are primitive.

4) Geographical distribution. If the group is widely distributed and has a recognisable centre or centres of diversity, i.e. areas where there are more species than elsewhere, then these centres may have been where the group first evolved. If so, the characters of the species in the centres of diversity will tend to show primitive states. The problem with this is that the group may have largely or completely died out in its centres of origin, so that subsequent areas of colonisation appear more prominent. In this case, character states will appear to be primitive which are in fact advanced. Therefore this cri-terion too is unreliable. There has been a good deal written on the relation of biogeography and cladistics, but the methods have not usually been objective enough to find expression as computer algorithms which will aid in the construction of taxon cladograms using information about distribution. Page (1988) has published a program for the opposite problem of constructing area cladograms.

5) Geological strata. If fossil material is available from strata of known geological age, then the primitive states occur in the oldest fossils. It is rarely possible to use this argument, except when fossils are available. Even then, there are problems since the fossil record may be incomplete.

3.3.4 Transformation rules

When reconstructing a tree of evolution, assumptions have to be made about *transformation rules*. These correspond roughly to assumptions about the rate of evolutionary change, whether this is equal in different lines, and whether reversals can occur. These rules affect the method which is used to construct trees, or to fit characters to trees. If incorrect assumptions are made about rates of evolutionary change, it is possible to deduce a wrong tree from correct character data (Felsenstein, 1978b).

A) The simplest assumption (Camin and Sokal, 1965) to make about changes in a character during evolution is that each can change only once, from primitive to advanced (0 to 1), and that changes in the opposite direction (1 to 0) do not occur. The number of these changes is then minimised.

B) Wagner parsimony (Kluge and Farris, 1969). Changes from advanced to primitive (1 to 0) are allowed as well as changes from 0 to 1. The total number of changes is then minimised.

C) Dollo parsimony (Le Quesne, 1974). Only one change from 0 to 1 per character is allowed, but as many changes from 1 to 0 are allowed as are needed to explain the data, and the number of these is minimised.

D) Polymorphism method (Felsenstein, 1979). Instead of insisting that each binary character in a taxon is invariable, it is permitted to vary, so that it may be either 0 or 1 (written as P). The transition from a primitive to a polymorphic state (0 to P) is allowed once per character. After that, a polymorphic character could persist for some time as new taxa evolve (P stays P) or a polymorphism could change back to primitive (P to 0), or a polymorphism could change to advanced (P to 1). The method then minimises the total length of the time periods in which polymorphisms endure, i.e. the number of P states on tree branches.

3.3.5 Algorithms for constructing cladograms

One of the difficulties which recurs in the construction of evolutionary trees is that many of the algorithms which are used lead to a large number of alternative hypothetical trees. In the absence of any other criterion, how should the 'right' tree be chosen? In this situation, the principle of *parsimony* is applied. The tree with the smallest number of character changes is preferred. This choice is simply an expediency in order to make the problem soluble. It is not based on any assumption to the effect that evolution did actually proceed by the most parsimonious or economical path. There is no reason to believe that this was so; indeed, to the contrary. Nothing more than Occam's Razor is being applied, namely that when you have numerous alternative hypotheses without any other reason for preference, the best option is to choose the simplest (shortest) solution. It quite often happens that even with this simplifying assumption, there are several alternative trees of minimum length. In this case, a subjective choice could be made, or it may be possible to form some composite or *consensus* tree from the features of the individual trees (Adams, 1972; Mickevich, 1978; Rohlf, 1982). Felsenstein (1984, 1985a) has investigated the statistical significance of trees of different lengths. In his example, which used 20 characters, he found no significant difference in the likelihood that a tree might be the 'right' tree in the range from the shortest tree up to trees which were 9 steps longer. This indicates that there is in fact little reason to regard the shortest tree as the best hypothesis. Felsenstein also comments that when there are several alternative trees of minimum length, a subgroup would have to occur in 95% of alternative trees before it would be sufficiently significant to merit inclusion in a consensus.

Once a starting set of assumptions and hypotheses has been chosen, as above, then there are three broad classes of algorithm which might be used to construct cladograms. The first two classes are analogous to the types of algorithms used for finding diagnostic descriptions, (p. 154). The classes are:

1) Complete search of all trees. This has the advantage that all the most parsimonious trees will be found, but the disadvantage that it can take a prohibitively long time except for small data sets. There do exist programming techniques which will cut down the searching needed, and which will cope with slightly larger data sets.

2) Heuristic search. A method which will search in a rational way for a reasonably short tree. This has the advantage of speed, but the disadvantage that there is no way of knowing whether the tree found is the best one, or whether there are others equally as good, or where they may be found.

3) Graphical search. A type of program which illustrates possible trees and the characters on them, and which provides tools for manipulating and exploring the trees. In a sense this approach does not provide an algorithm at all, but is more a computer-aided means of searching by hand.

An example of a heuristic algorithm is that described by Farris (1970), which is related to the so-called groundplan divergence algorithm of Wagner (1963). The characters of the taxa are coded as 0 for primitive and 1 for advanced. If an ordered tree is wanted, then designate the ancestor as a base taxon. This could be either a real taxon or a hypothetical one. If an unordered method is wanted, then one taxon is selected arbitrarily as a base. Thereafter the distances between all the taxa and the base are calculated. The distance between two taxa is zero for a character if they have the same state, or 1 if they are different, and this is summed over all characters. Find the taxon which is closest to the base, call it A, and attach it to the tree. The first time, this just means creating a branch from base to A. The next time, the next unplaced taxon which is closest to the base is selected (B, say) and it is added to the tree. This may be done either by adding B to an existing node, or by creating a hypothetical taxon in the middle of an existing branch and attaching B to that. The various possibilities are examined and the most parsimonious arrangement is adopted. If there is a tie and there is more than one arrangement which is equally efficient, then one of them is chosen arbitrarily. The process is repeated until all taxa have been placed and the tree or network is complete. There is still a stage of optimisation needed after the tree is made. The details of this will not be described here, but the effect of it is to reassign the hypothetical taxa which were invented during the first stage so as to be sure that they optimise the tree. This algorithm produces one tree (unless ties are exploited) and this tree is not necessarily the most parsimonious possible. If different hypothetical ancestors are tried as a starting point, then other trees may also be found. Notice that the transformation rule assumed is type B, Wagner parsimony (see above). The algorithm as just described does not allow for the possibility that any of the extant taxa might be ancestral to others, or to put it another way, existing taxa can only occur at the tips of the branches of the cladogram. In the algorithm of Wagner (1963) it was possible to have existing taxa at internal nodes of the cladogram.

An extension of Farris' algorithm is used by Swofford (1983) in the PAUP program, such that branches are swapped around at various stages of the tree-building process in the hope of finding better solutions. This of course increases the time taken, and the algorithm performs something more like a complete search.

Using the example of the genus *Epilobium* and the subset of data in Table 3.6, the PAUP program was used to produce the cladogram in Fig. 3.12. For 6 species and 10 characters, 4 slightly differing cladograms were produced,

Table 3.6 Reduced *Epilobium* matrix for cladistics

Primitive state = 1, advanced states = 2(3), ? variable.

Taxon		Characters									
		4	5	7	9	10	11	14	15	16	17
0. ANCESTOR	X	1	1	1	1	1	1	1	1	1	1
3. montanum	C	1	1	2	1	2	1	2	2	1	1
4. lanceolatum	D	1	2	2	1	1	1	2	2	1	1
5. roseum	E	2	2	2	1	1	1	1	1	2	2
6. ciliatum	F	2	2	2	1	2	1	2	1	1	2
7. tetragonum	G	1	2	1	2	1	2	2	1	2	1
9. obscurum	I	1	2	1	2	2	1	3	1	2	2
10. palustre	J	1	1	1	1	1	1	2	1	1	1

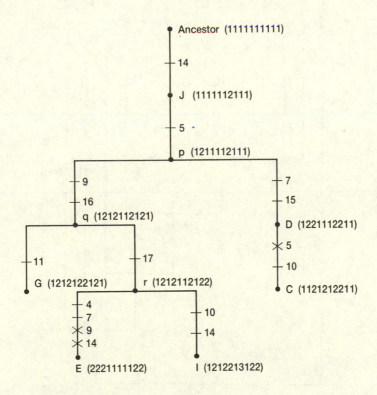

Ancestor (1111111111)

+ 14

J (1111112111)

+ 5

p (1211112111)

+ 9
+ 16
q (1212112121)

+ 7
+ 15
D (1221112211)

× 5
+ 10
C (1121212211)

+ 11
G (1212122121)

+ 17
r (1212112122)

+ 4
+ 7
× 9
× 14
E (2221111122)

+ 10
+ 14
I (1212213122)

+ change from primitive to advanced.

× reversal, advanced to primitive.
    Character nos. which change are shown on branches.
    Character states shown in brackets.
    p, q, r are hypothetical taxa.

Fig. 3.12 An *Epilobium* cladogram from Table 3.6.

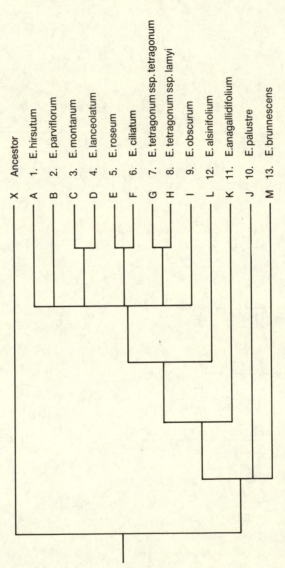

Fig. 3.13 Adam's consensus cladogram for *Epilobium* trial A.

all of the same length. This cladogram has 4 reversals of character state, and includes three hypothetical taxa. Another run with the complete data matrix of 13 species gave 41 rather similar trees all with the same length of 47 steps. An Adam's consensus of these 41 trees is illustrated in Fig. 3.13. The process was repeated with different assumptions for the polarity of character states. For the first trial (trial A), the ancestor was given the states coded as 1's. Trial B took the completely opposite assumption, with the ancestor coded with states 2 or 3, and this gave 57 trees, still of length 47. Lastly, in trial C, the ancestor was coded with alternate states 1 or 2/3, giving over 100 trees. The species groupings for these three trials, and their predictivities, are shown in Table 3.4. The predictivity for trial A is the best, although not nearly as good as that for the best phenetic arrangement, but for trials B and C it is much lower. It appears that quite different cladograms with quite different predictivity will result from different assumptions about character polarity. As noted above, there is no way of constructing a cladogram without reversals for this data as it stands, i.e. homoplasy cannot be avoided. The characters and their polarity can be now be reconsidered with a view to finding a better arrangement which leads to a shorter tree. If characters are added or removed, or polarities changed, to get a better theory, then well and good. However, it is important to realise that success in obtaining a satisfactory cladogram is not a proof, as is sometimes claimed, that the initial assumptions about choice of characters, polarity and ancestors or outgroups were correct; all that can be said is that the results will be consistent with the starting assumptions.

The computational problem of searching for the most direct evolutionary trees belongs to a general class of what are known as combinatorial problems, i.e. where there are a large number of alternatives to be examined. There is a general method for coping with such problems known as the *branch and bound* technique. The idea is that sections of the problem can be identified where it can be shown that there is a group of cases which are not worth looking at. In the case of evolutionary trees, it is sometimes possible to know that all the trees which can be obtained by manipulating a given tree whose length is known are going to be as long or longer than that. Hence there is no point in searching that particular group of trees. A mathematical explanation of this is given by Hendy and Penny (1982). A branch and bound algorithm is provided in some of the cladistic programs, e.g. PAUP, and enables somewhat larger problems to be examined than would otherwise be the case. Nevertheless, these complete search algorithms are still limited to relatively small groups of taxa, and it is time to explore the reasons for this.

3.3.6 The number of possible evolutionary trees

Let us suppose to begin with that the data matrix contains only binary characters. This means that the branches of any evolutionary tree based on it will all be two-way forks. If the tips of the branches correspond with known taxa, then these are said to be labelled. The other (internal) nodes of the tree will correspond to hypothetical taxa which do not have to fit with known taxa, and these are said to be unlabelled nodes. For the case of a rooted binary tree with unlabelled interior nodes and with labelled tips, Felsenstein (1978a) gives a formula for the number of possible trees for n taxa, which is

$$\text{The product from } k = 2 \text{ to } n \text{ of} \quad (2k-3) \;=\; \frac{(2n-3)!}{2^{n-2}(n-2)!}$$

If the interior nodes are labelled, i.e. they correspond to known fossil ancestors, the number of possible trees is

$$n^{n-1}$$

which is an even larger number. Also, if multiway branches are allowed in the tree with unlabelled interior nodes, the number of possible trees is again greater. The top formula gives a rate of increase in the number of trees which is worse than exponential but not as bad as n to the power $n-1$. These formulae do not convey very much by themselves, but a comparison of figures is given in Table 3.7. This makes it very clear why it is impractical to use a complete search algorithm, even using branch and bound, for anything much over about 20 taxa. To put it another way, if your program in your computer found the shortest tree for 20 taxa in say, 10 minutes, then to find the shortest tree

Table 3.7 Comparison of numbers of trees

n	exponential	formula	n^{n-1}
1	1	1	1
2	2	1	2
3	4	3	9
4	8	15	64
5	16	105	625
6	32	945	7776
7	64	10395	117649
8	128	135135	2097152
9	256	2027025	43046721
10	512	34459425	1000000000
20	131072	8.2×10^{21}	5.24×10^{24}
100	2.1×10^9	3.35×10^{184}	10^{198}

for 100 taxa, which is a realistic size of problem, would take about 6×10^{179} years (compare with the estimated age of the universe, about 2×10^{10} years!). The only thing which could be done is to divide a larger group of taxa into smaller groups, if suitable synapomorphies can be found, and then to combine the resulting trees afterwards. Unfortunately, it is well known that in this kind of problem, joining suboptimal partial trees does not lead to a global optimum, and there would be no reason to believe that the result would be parsimonious. Alternatively, it may be possible to calculate a least upper boundary for the minimum size of tree. This has been done for other similar problems. However, unless we knew how far the boundary would be from the true minimum this would be no help.

The problem of searching for the most direct evolutionary tree belongs to a general class of computational problems known as the *NP-complete problems*, whose mathematical properties have been studied extensively. A mathematical proof that this problem belongs to this class is given by Graham and Foulds (1982). NP-completeness is not very difficult to understand, in spite of its peculiar name. A very readable explanation of it is given by Lewis and Papadimitriou (1978). Mathematicians have studied the time it takes for a computer to solve certain kinds of combinatorial problems with N cases. This time always increases with N, as expected. Some problems have the property that the time needed increases as some polynomial function of N, such as the square or the cube, for example. This may sound like a steep increase, but if we consider the example given above of the rise from 20 to 100 cases, this is only an increase of say, 25 to 600 times. This puts up the time from 10 minutes to say, 100 hours, which is still practicable, if the solution to the problem is really important. The really difficult problems are those for which the rate of time increase is *non-polynomial*. This is what the letters NP stand for. The time for an NP-problem may be quite reasonable up to a certain value of N, but in all cases it reaches a point where the further rate of rise is astronomical, as with our previous example. In other words, such problems become totally impractical beyond a certain point, such that any amount of time or any imaginable increase of computer speed would not help. Interestingly, it has been shown that many of the NP-problems belong to a more general class of problems known as *NP-complete* problems. These have the property such that, if an effective algorithm to any one of these problems were found, then this solution would also apply to all the rest. Intriguingly, although this has been done for some other kinds of problem, it has not been possible to prove that the solution to the NP-complete class of problem does not exist. Nevertheless, mathematicians and computer experts have laboured for many years to find a solution, without success. It looks like one of those mathematical problems, like Fermat's Last Theorem, for which a solution may never be found. All the same, if a solution could be found, it would be of enormous practical value, quite apart from the particular kind of problem which has been of interest here.

3.3.7 Compatibility analysis

This term applies to a different class of methods where the aim is to avoid homoplasy at the outset. If the sets of characters which are used to construct cladograms are mutually compatible (a clique) then homoplasy is absent. Meacham (1980) gives details of the method. Characters may be compatible for spurious reasons, as for example when one character is logically or functionally dependent on another. The same arguments apply here as given above for choosing evolutionary characters. Meacham (1984) describes statistical experiments to discover whether compatibility of characters might be due to chance or to evolution. As with the methods described earlier, it is not necessary to know the polarity of the characters unless a tree is desired. A network of relations between taxa can be created and a root chosen for it later.

In the present context, a *true* character is one whose distribution of states corresponds to the actual tree of evolution. It is not possible to know which the true characters are, but it is possible to identify sets of characters which cannot be true all at once. Statements about character compatibility are facts and not hypotheses.

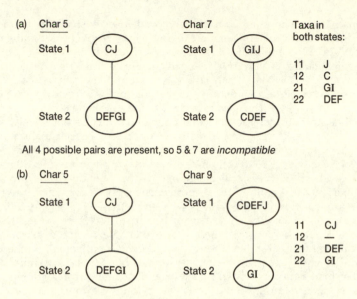

(a)   Char 5

State 1   CJ

State 2   DEFGI

Char 7

State 1   GIJ

State 2   CDEF

Taxa in
both states:

11	J
12	C
21	GI
22	DEF

All 4 possible pairs are present, so 5 & 7 are *incompatible*

(b)   Char 5

State 1   CJ

State 2   DEFGI

Char 9

State 1   CDEFJ

State 2   GI

11	CJ
12	—
21	DEF
22	GI

Only 3 of the possible pairs of states occur, so 5 & 9 are *compatible*

Fig. 3.14   Recognising compatible characters in *Epilobium*.

In order to decide whether two characters are compatible or not, it is not necessary to try and draw cladograms with them. A simple method is illustrated in Fig. 3.14. In diagram a, characters 5 and 7 are compared from the subset of *Epilobium* data in Table 3.6. The letters in the balloons represent lists of the taxa which have states 1 and 2. Next, make a table of all the possible character-state pairs which can be formed from two binary characters with states 1 and 2. There are four of these, 11, 12, 21 and 22. In the table, list the taxa which occur in both balloons, e.g. for 11, the taxa are CJ for character 5 state 1 and GIJ for character 7 state 1, so the list of common taxa (exclusive 'or') is just taxon J. Repeat this for the other 3 pairs. If all 4 entries in the table are non-empty, then the characters are incompatible. Conversely, if there is a line in this table which is empty, the characters are compatible. Hence characters 5 and 7 are incompatible. In diagram b, it turns out that there are no taxa in the 12 lines of the table, so therefore characters 5 and 9 are compatible. Another way of looking at this is to compare the balloons, one from each character, which contain the shortest taxon list, i.e. the least common state for each character. If the smaller set of taxa is completely included in the larger, if they are identical, or if the two sets are disjoint, i.e. do not share a common taxon at all, then the two characters are compatible.

The method continues by combining compatible pairs of characters into larger groups (cliques). The algorithm searches for the largest clique or cliques, since there may be several of the maximum size. The largest clique is then a reasonable choice of characters, and this can be used to draw a cladogram without homoplasy, which is the best hypothesis. It often happens that there are several cliques of the same maximum size, so some choice or consensus has to be made between them. It may also happen that the characters in the maximal clique are inadequate for resolving the cladogram.

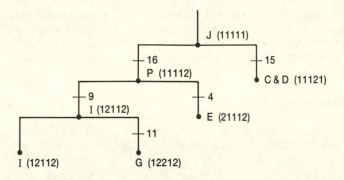

P   is a hypothetical taxon

+   represents character change from primitive
to advanced (reversals do not occur)

Fig. 3.15 Cladogram from compatibility analysis of 5 *Epilobium* characters.

If the maximal clique is found to be unsatisfactory for some reason, then it is possible to continue the analysis to a second stage. The characters which are common to all the maximal cliques will also form a compatible set. A network can be formed with this intersecting set. There are characters which occurred in the maximal cliques which are left out of this reduced network. Next, break this network at some node and try to add some of the omitted characters to each part. If this is successful, the result will be a larger network, on which most of the characters are compatible, but where some characters will only be compatible in part of the network.

The CLINCH program due to G.F. Estabrook and K.Fiala (Fiala, 1984) was used to examine the *Epilobium* data of Table 3.6. The program found 6 cliques all of the same size, with 5 characters each. All 6 cliques were unsatisfactory because in each case, there were not sufficient characters available to distinguish all the taxa from each other, so that no clique was completely resolved. A cladogram based on one of these is shown in Fig. 3.15, arbitrarily chosen to resemble that in Fig. 3.12. Other cladograms could have been chosen which are not so similar.

3.3.8 Available program packages

Comments on the features and performance of various computer programs tend to go out of date extremely quickly, so no detailed review will be attempted (but see Fink, 1986 and Platnick, 1987). There are a number of popular programs which will construct parsimonious cladograms from data matrices, such as PAUP (Swofford, 1983), PHYLIP (Felsenstein, 1985a,b), HENNIG86 (Farris, 1988) and MacClade (Maddison and Maddison, 1987). PHYLIP, PAUP and HENNIG86 offer both heuristic and exhaustive (branch and bound) algorithms, which will cope with both ordered and unordered trees, offer a variety of different transformation rules, and provide various utilities for drawing trees. MacClade is different in that it provides an interactive graphic display of different trees and characters, which can be manipulated in order to explore various alternatives, without including very much by way of algorithms for searching for trees. CLINCH (Fiala, 1984) is a program for compatibility analysis.

3.3.9 Summary

The use of cladistic methods requires a number of assumptions or approximations and subjective decisions to be made. These may be summarised as follows.

1)   That a tree based on actual or supposed genealogy is the best way to represent relationships between taxa. Evidently hypothetical relationships of ancestry will be well represented, but other kinds of relationship may or may not be represented accurately, so this is dubious.

2)   It is assumed that it is possible to know which taxa belong to a monophyletic group. The same assumption is made about out- or sister-groups.

3)   It is assumed that it is possible to know which characters reflect evolutionary history, and which do not, and that the changes in the states of these characters correspond to evolutionary events. The latter assumption is known to be incorrect if hybridisation has taken place, which is often the case for plants. Characters which show states which do not fit this assumption (homoplasy) are quite common.

4)   It is assumed that it is possible to know which are the primitive and advanced states of characters.

5)   Assumptions have to be made about whether character state reversals can take place, and how often, and whether the rates of evolution in different taxa at different times are the same or different. These assumptions express themselves in different transformation rules.

6)   The assumption of parsimony is not correct; it is merely a simplification. Even so, there is reason to doubt whether the most parsimonious trees are statistically significant.

These six assumptions are often very approximate. Even after that, there are a number of practical problems:

1)   The algorithms do not cope well with variable (polymorphic) or numerical characters.

2)   The algorithms for finding trees are either heuristic, i.e. they are reasonably rapid, but do not provide a complete answer, or are complete but quite impractical for larger data sets. There is no generally satisfactory way of finding the most parsimonious trees.

3)   Even when the shortest trees have been found, it often turns out that there are a number of differing trees of equal size. It may be possible to combine these with a consensus method, but the trees need to be very similar before this can be done with confidence, which is often not the case.

The existing algorithms for constructing cladograms do not provide a general-purpose practical method to solve the problem of how to reconstruct evolutionary history. The algorithms might perform better if more character data were available, i.e. more characters with better consistency, such that fewer alternative cladograms are produced, and with a better consensus. This difficulty has long been recognised by taxonomists even before the advent of the modern computer methods. It seems unlikely that more and better data will come from the morphology of organisms. Biochemical molecular data may provide a better source of data in the future. It also seems very likely that improvement on the computational side can only be obtained if algorithms of a radically different kind can be found.

There has been much controversy about phenetic versus evolutionary methods of classification, and the question has often been asked, which type of method should be used? Since each type of method has different aims and different kinds of classification result, a student ought to experiment with both types of methods. It must be borne in mind, however, that the phenetic methods involve few subjective decisions, do not involve any major approximations and have effective algorithms. On the other hand, the cladistic methods are much more ambitious, involve many subjective decisions and several major approximations, and do not have generally effective algorithms.

4

Conventional
identification methods

In this chapter, all identification methods which make no use of calculation
or computers are discussed. These are, broadly speaking, the methods most
used up to the present time: the diagnostic key, the multi-access key, and the
comparison method.

The discussion in this chapter, and elsewhere, is unified to some extent by
the repeated use of the same example, the British species of the higher plant
genus *Epilobium*. The descriptive data in Fig. 1.1 are largely derived from
Clapham, Tutin and Warburg (1962). For non-botanists, such technical terms
as are used are defined below Fig. 1.1; Figs. 1.2 to 1.5 and 4.2 were all derived
from Fig. 1.1 by the author.

4.1 Diagnostic keys

4.1.1 Use

There are two principal kinds of key: *the parallel* (or *bracketed)* style, as in Fig.
1.4, and the *yoked* (or *indented*) style, as in Fig. 1.5 The term 'indented' is
unfortunate, because indentation could be used in the layout of either kind.
The essential difference is that in the parallel variety, all the components of a
set of related questions are printed together, whereas in the yoked kind, all the
possibilities which depend on part of a question are set down and exhausted
first before other parts of a question are taken up. For example in Fig. 1.4
(parallel), the two kinds of 'leaf stalk length', i.e. 'sessile' or 'stalked', appear
together as the components of the question labelled 6. On the other hand, in
Fig. 1.5 (yoked), the first part of question 6 (leaves sessile) is fully explored,
down to the question labelled 8, before the alternative (leaves stalked) is taken
up again. These alternative parts of questions in keys are called *leads* or *legs*
(because they lead from one question to another).

Before discussing how to use a key, one needs to consider the matter of
finding or choosing a key. Often the identity of a specimen in the wider
sense is already known, e.g. there may be no difficulty in knowing that one
has an insect, or a fern. If the class, order or family is uncertain, there exist
keys for these broad categories, e.g. for families of angiosperms (flowering
plants), (Davis and Cullen, 1965), or for orders of insects in the world (Brues
et al., 1954). Textbooks on taxonomy contain general advice on identification,
e.g. for plants (Lawrence, 1951), for animals (Mayr, 1969) and for microbes

(Cowan and Steel, 1965). It may be possible to find a key which is restricted to the appropriate geographical area, so that there is no need to consider taxa which are not known to occur in the area of origin of the specimen. Even if there is no such key, there may exist a check list of known taxa from the area in question, and this can be used in conjunction with a more generalised key to help eliminate some of the possibilities.

Let us illustrate the use of a key with Fig. 1.4 (a parallel key). We have a specimen of a plant to identify. There must be some reason for choosing to use this key, i.e. we are assuming that the plant is (a) from the genus *Epilobium* (possibly by using a generic key before), and (b) that it is one of those included in this key (e.g. because it came from the appropriate geographical area). If we are confident that these conditions are met, then begin at the top with the question labelled 1 at the left, i.e. does the stem root at the nodes, etc? Suppose the answer is no, and the stem is erect, then the number of the next question is shown at the far right, i.e. 2. Refer now to question 2, i.e. is the stem terete (round) or does it have raised lines? If raised lines are present, we lead on to question 6. Continuing this process, assuming that the specimen has stalked leaves, and glandular hairs on the stem, and leaf rounded at base, we arrive at the second lead of question 10. At the right there is the name of a species *(ciliatum)* instead of the number of a further question. Our specimen has 'keyed out' to *E. ciliatum*. To be sure this is right, check the characters given in the rest of the lead (if any), and then look up a complete description of the taxon and compare, or else compare it with named museum specimens, line drawings or photographs, as convenient. The identification should usually also agree with one's previous experience, and fit in with knowledge of geographical distribution and of seasonality.

What happens if neither of the alternatives to a lead agrees exactly? As an example, consider once again question 10 in Fig. 1.4. Suppose that the specimen has leaf cuneate at base, petals pink, and stigma less than style. Neither *E.roseum* or *E.ciliatum* is exactly like that. However, out of the three characters asked for, the former agrees with one of three and the latter with two. On a majority vote therefore, *E.ciliatum* is more nearly correct, and that would be the tentative conclusion. If the characters were split equally between the two sides of the couplet, then you would either have to make a subjective choice by giving certain characters more importance, or explore both alternatives.

The use of the yoked key of Fig. 1.5 is little different from this. Since the two leads of question 2 are not printed together, we have to look down the page for the alternative leads. This is why the questions are indented, so as to make the related leads easier to find. The last lead of a question is marked with an asterisk, so that none is overlooked in cases where there are more than two. Once we have chosen a lead, e.g. 'stem with raised lines', the next question is immediately in the next line, i.e. number 6, 'leaves more or less sessile'.

What has been said so far about using a key has assumed that there were no errors in the recognition of characters of the specimen. Suppose however, using the above example again, that we really did have a specimen of *E. ciliatum*, but erroneously thought that its leaves were sessile, leading to question 7. Here the second lead fits much better than the first, although the flower diameter is not correct. This then leads to 8, and 'leaf rounded at base' suggests *obscurum*. A check with a flora should show that this is wrong, because the stem of *obscurum* has no glandular hairs, whereas *ciliatum* has, besides differences of flower size and colour (see Fig. 1.1). Failure to check might result in the mistake passing unnoticed! Once the mistake is recognised one can return to the key and work back from the lead for *E.obscurum*, and ask which character might have been wrong, and when a mistake is found, work forwards through the key again to another answer. It is often said that the yoked type of key is better for working backwards in this situation, because the previous lead, which pointed to the current one, is always on the line above. However a parallel key can easily be provided with the lead numbers of previous questions. In Fig. 1.4, these are provided in brackets after the question numbers on the left.

Another situation where errors can arise is when the specimen is of a taxon not included in the key. It might be a new species, a non-native or a hybrid, or, most likely, belong to another genus or family altogether. Once again, it is possible to work right through the key without noticing anything wrong, unless the tentative identification is checked afterwards. Incongruities in characters can occur which will show up this situation. For example, in question 2 of the *Epilobium* key, 'stem terete' (rounded in cross-section) is compared with 'stem with raised lines'. If the specimen had a square stem, an error would at once be suspected.

Suppose that one were not sure whether the leaves had stalks or not. One could temporise, by trying all outcomes of question 6, i.e. questions 7 and 9; but if question 7 again raises a doubt, confusion is soon reached. This illustrates a fundamental fault of the key as an identification method; namely, that it requires the use of specified characters which may not be available or convenient. To some extent, this difficulty can be avoided by providing alternative keys, e.g. for flowering and fruiting material, or for male as well as female insects, but it is impossible to construct a diagnostic key which will meet every situation.

4.1.2 Construction

Any key has to be based on a knowledge of characters and their corresponding states. This is obtained by examining living organisms, preserved specimens and taxonomic handbooks. There are hazards even in this process, since specimens (living or preserved) may not be correctly identified, and different authors may not use the same definitions of taxa, or may be using the same descriptive terms with different meanings.

The size of the group should be considered, as keys to more than one or two hundred taxa tend to be unwieldy. A good way to deal with a large group is to subdivide it with an initial key, using only very carefully chosen characters, which then direct the user to subsidiary keys, e.g. as in the key to Angiosperm families in Clapham *et al.* (1962). Very large keys do exist however; the longest known to the author has 2117 leads and is again to Angiosperm families, by Geesink *et al.* (1981).

The different characters, once obtained, will differ in their usefulness for making keys. In what follows, a 'good' character means one which is good for making keys, and is not necessarily useful for other purposes. An assessment of the 'goodness' of characters is often called *character weighting*. This may be expressed as a preference, or numerically. Good characters have various aspects:

(i) *Ease of observation*. Characters which can be seen with the unaided eye will always be more practical to observe than those requiring special equipment, e.g. microscopy or chemical tests. Under this heading also come questions of availability of characters, e.g. for a species with two sexes a character which occurs on both is better. Similarly, for preserved specimens, colours are often lost and some characters are seasonal in their appearance, e.g. those of the fruit of plants.

(ii) *Information content*. Suppose there are 10 species in a genus, of which five show a certain state of a character and five show another. This is then a very informative character for separating species. On the other hand, states in the proportion of 1 to 9 denote a character which gives little information. Such a character may be highly *diagnostic* for a particular species, but is little use for distinguishing species in general. Another way to put this is that a character which is very variable *between* species is highly informative. On the other hand, a character which varies greatly *within* species and whose states overlap, is very little use for distinguishing taxa and carries little information. Finally, a character which is constant throughout the genus has no information content at all, except for defining the genus, but might be useful for distinguishing it from other genera. The information content of a character has meaning only in relation to the taxa which are being considered, and is not an absolute concept.

The definition of characters and states which are being used may be perfectly evident from standard usage, but if any terms are being used in a non-standard way, or if specialised characters occur which apply only to the organisms in question, then it is important to supply definitions. For the example which follows, definitions are supplied under Fig. 1.1 Some well chosen line drawings or illustrations may be very helpful here.

Characters can be of different types. A *qualitative* character is simply a statement, such as 'shape of head' whereas a *quantitative* character concerns a number or a measurement, e.g. 'number of legs', 'height of stem'. Quantitative characters may be *discrete*, e.g. 'number of petals' or *continuous*, e.g. 'length of wing'. Continuous quantitative characters tend to show a great deal of variation, mostly due to environmental influences on the growth of organisms, and are therefore often poor characters from the point of view of information content.

It might seem unnecessary to point out that states of characters used in keys have to be *contrasting*, or *mutually exclusive*, were it not for the number of examples available where this rule is broken. For example, suppose the character 'petal colour' has been given three states, 'red', 'blue' and 'spotted'. There are really two characters here, namely: 'colour of petal' (= red or blue) and 'distribution of petal colour' (= uniform, or spotted). A way to detect this failure to contrast is to ask whether any two states can apply simultaneously, e.g. can petals be 'red' and 'spotted' at the same time? They can, so these states are not exclusive and do not contrast. If states which are not exclusive of each other are used in a key, it may be impossible to decide which lead to take. Not only must states be mutually exclusive, so must leads. For example,

Wings present, 5-12 mm long
Wings absent or present, and if present, 8-20 mm long

will be useless for a winged specimen with wings 10 mm long.

The starting point for the construction of any key is a rectangular table of the taxa and their characters. This is also called a *data matrix*, and an example is shown in Fig. 1.1. There may be a number of gaps in the table where characters are missing. The reason for this may be simply that the table is based on a source which did not contain all the information. The source would have been more useful for this purpose if the information had been complete, because greater flexibility in key construction would then have been possible. Another reason why characters may not be scored is that it may be impossible to score them. For example, if insects in a group can be winged or wingless, then 'shape of wing' is a character which is irrelevant for wingless species. This is called a *conditional* or *dependent* character.

Which type of key is to be preferred, parallel or yoked? The former may take slightly less space in publications, because no room is taken up for indentation. If suitably presented, they are both equally suited to back-tracking for errors. The yoked type is said to be less convenient when it comes to finding contrasting leads, but this can be mitigated by providing marginal notes to show where the next lead is (if it is on another page), and whether it is the final lead of its kind. On the other hand, the yoked type can show the relationships between species, in so far as a key is a suitable way of doing this. It has already been argued (p. 9) that this consideration is not relevant. Hence there is very little difference in merit on technical grounds between the two kinds of key, although there may be subjective preferences. This viewpoint is rather in contrast with that of other authors, who frequently argue strongly for one kind or the other.

We now come to the construction of an actual key. To begin with, choose a character which is easy to observe and understand, and which divides the species into two groups of as nearly as possible equal size. The advantage of equal branching is that it tends to produce a key with the smallest average number of questions required to reach each taxon; with fewer questions, other things being equal, there are fewer chances of error. The character should also show as little variation within taxa as possible. If it is not possible to satisfy all these rules at once, it is suggested that ease of observation should take precedence.

These points will be illustrated from the data matrix shown in Fig. 1.1 and the keys of Figs. 1.4 and 1.5. Which characters are easy to observe? This means those which can be assessed with the unaided eye, and which will be observable regardless of the condition of the specimen, i.e. in this example, with or without flowers or fruit, and living or preserved. If we assume that the plant has stem and leaves at least but not necessarily flowers or fruit, characters 5, 7, 9 and 10 could be a first choice. Which of these is best distributed? Character 10 (leaf base shape) is best, with 6 taxa in one state and 7 in the other. Next comes 5 (stem lines) with taxa in the ratio of 4 to 9. Character 7 is a little variable and character 9 is missing in many cases, so dismiss these. Although character 10 is better distributed, its two states are not very clearly distinct, so character 5 will be preferred as a starting character.

In fact, however, the example keys begin with quite a different character, illustrating another principle. If there exist taxa which are strikingly different from the others, it is often convenient to dispose of these first, at or near the beginning of the key. Some authors strongly recommend this procedure as a desirable feature of key making. It may not always be a matter of choice since, if there are taxa which really are very distinct from the others, it is quite likely that they will show states which contrast in characters which are chosen near the beginning of the key. In other words, it may be that the only convenient way to make a key involves distinguishing 'unusual' taxa first. In the example there is one highly distinct species, *E. brunnescens*, which has a creeping and rooting stem, unlike all the rest, so this is keyed out first. There is no necessity to do this in this instance, as other keys could be made which leave *E. brunnescens* to appear later.

Examination of Fig. 1.1 will show that *E. brunnescens* is the only species to have the character states 'prostrate' for character 1, and 'stem rooting at nodes', as opposed to 'not rooting' for character 6. These characters are diagnostic for this species as they are unique to it, and are alone sufficient to identify it. There is in fact another diagnostic character for this species, flower position (12). This is not so useful as the others as flowers might not be available, but it is put in as an *auxiliary character*. It is another piece of information which could help to confirm the other distinctions made in lead 1 of the key.

So far we have chosen leads 1 and 2. One taxon has been eliminated. Considering the first part of lead 2, 'stem more or less terete', we can temporarily dismiss any taxa which do not have this character state, leaving just four taxa, i.e. numbers 1 to 3 and 10. Which characters can now be used? Only those which still show some variation among this group of taxa. Looking only at columns 1 to 3 and 10 in Fig. 1.1, one finds that only characters 3, 4, 8, 10, 13, 14 and 15 show any differences between taxa, characters 1, 6, 12 and 18 are the same for each, characters 9, 11, 16, 17 are incomplete or missing, and characters 2 and 7 are rather variable. Of the first group, characters 3, 4 and 10 divide the four taxa neatly into two pairs, and are leaf and stem characters. Character 10 has states which are not very distinct, so that is dismissed again. Both characters 3 and 4 require the use of a hand lens, but are clear cut. However, character 3 ('direction of stem hairs') is a conditional character depending on whether the stem has simple hairs, and in fact three out of four of the taxa can at times be 'glabrous' (without simple hairs). Hence character 4 ('presence of glandular hairs') is chosen for lead 3.

Now that lead 3 has been established, auxiliary characters can be sought to add to it. If there are other characters whose states are distributed in the *same way* as the states of character 4, these could be used to confirm the division. This is not quite the same situation as in lead 1, where the auxiliary characters were also diagnostic characters. Characters 3, 8, 10, and 13 to 15 are the possibles but only 3 has the right distribution. Hence lead 3 could be written:

3 Stem with glandular hairs and spreading simple hairs.
  Stem without glandular hairs, with appressed simple hairs.

However, simple hairs may not be present, so it would be better to put:

3 Stem with glandular hairs; simple hairs, if present, spreading.
  Stem without glandular hairs; simple hairs, if present, appressed.

If information was available about the frequency of plants with or without simple hairs, the following might be better:

3 Stem with glandular hairs, usually with spreading simple hairs.
  Stem without glandular hairs, glabrous or with appressed simple hairs.

This auxiliary character is now logically correct, but less straightforward than it might have been, since it is now qualified by doubt ('usually') and with an alternative ('or'). Since characters in keys ought to be easy to understand, it can be argued that this auxiliary character is more complicated than useful. In the example keys, it has in fact been left out for this reason. Characters of habitat and distribution can be used as auxiliary characters, but should not be used elsewhere in keys, on account of the possibility that an organism can always be found in a new habitat or locality.

Continuing the process of building the key, the first part of lead 3 concerns just two taxa, *parviflorum* and *hirsutum*. Hence lead 4 is concerned just with listing differences between the two taxa, which 'key out' here, and terminates the branching of this part of the key. It may not necessarily be a good idea to use all the distinguishing and diagnostic characters at this point, but only those which are most striking, for if many characters are available, the result may just be an essay describing a taxon, which is better placed elsewhere.

The construction of the remainder of the key continues in the same manner until all taxa have been separated. It is usual practice to put the shorter leads of branches first when writing out a key. For example, the first part of branch 2 has two other branches depending on it and following it (3 and 4), whereas the second part has seven (6 to 12). The sole purpose of this is to reduce the distance which the eye has to travel down the page when moving to the later leads of the same question. Although the example keys are strictly *dichotomous* (with all leads in pairs), there is no strict logical necessity for this. Dichotomous keys are strongly preferred by many authors, especially in the yoked form, because of the possibility that if there are more than two leads in a question, the later ones could be overlooked. A key which includes *polytomous* questions (with more than two leads) may nonetheless be a more sensible choice in some cases, where characters are best expressed with many states. With *Epilobium,* a key to flowering plants could start with flower colour, but this has three states, so that the first question might say:

    1 Petals white to pale pink   roseum
      Petals rose   2
      Petals pink   3
This could be expressed just as well as a dichotomy like this:
    1 Petals white to pale pink   roseum
      Petals pink or rose   2
or as:
    1 Petals white to pale pink   roseum
      Petals coloured otherwise   2

which is not so good, because the use of 'otherwise' does not make clear what the alternatives are. If, for example, the specimen had 'petals blue', it would not be obvious that something was wrong. Another way of avoiding a polytomous character is to split it into a sequence of binary characters, e.g. 'petals pink or not pink', 'white to pale or not', 'rose or not', which is clumsy, and not recommended.

Another aspect of key construction is that of *taxon weighting*. This is the situation where one or more taxa are so frequently met with that it is desired to use as few questions as possible before these taxa are recognised. To put this another way, the length of the path through the key to such taxa is to be as short as possible, in order to save effort whenever a specimen of such a taxon is being identified. This is not the same situation as that for the 'unusual' taxon, because the common taxa may not have any particularly diagnostic characters. In order to write a key with weighted taxa, one must attempt to distinguish those taxa first, and so characters will be chosen in order to separate these taxa in particular rather than all taxa in general. Hence there may be some compromise with the general principles for key construction.

One may normally expect that a key can be used to separate every taxon concerned from every other. Indeed, if not, this could be a warning signal that the classification of the group is inadequate. In special cases, where a key is intended, say, for immature or preserved specimens only, there may be taxa which are not distinguishable with available characters, and then a *partial key* can be made up. The ultimate leads of such a key may give the names of more than one taxon, instead of one only. When such a key is in use, one may find that it is only possible to reach a short list of alternative identifications instead of a definitive one.

It may happen that a character varies in one taxon and not in another in such a way that the two taxa are neither distinct nor identical. For example, *E.hirsutum* always has a hairy stem, whereas *E.parviflorum* can be either glabrous or hairy. If this were the only character available, and a specimen has a glabrous stem, then it must be *E.parviflorum*, but if it has a hairy stem, then it is impossible to tell. This is called a *relative difference*. On the other hand *E.alsinifolium* always has a glabrous stem while *hirsutum* is hairy, and this is an *absolute difference*. A key could be continued to take advantage of a relative difference, which will allow some specimens to be recognised, by writing something like:

Stem glabrous	E.parviflorum
Stem hairy	E.hirsutum or E.parviflorum

Although in the example discussed above, variable and missing characters were given very little weight and were hardly used, there are times when they have to be used for lack of any alternative. The procedure then is to allow such a taxon to key out in more than one place. If there was an *Epilobium* species which could have leaves with or without stalks which belonged under the second part of lead 2 ('stem with raised lines'), then it would have to appear under both the leads labelled 6. Also, if these two character states are known to be easy to confuse in this taxon, one could deliberately put in both cases to reduce the chances of error. Likewise, if the state of this character was simply not known, and as there are two possible states, it could be treated in the same way. However, a character state which is inapplicable must not be treated like this, since it can never occur anyhow. It is recommended that missing or variable character states are used only sparingly, and are best avoided if possible. This is because they increase the total length of the key, especially if used at the beginning. To put this another way, they have less information content than constant or complete characters and tend therefore to be less useful.

If the organisms for which a key is wanted are polymorphic, there ought to be a separate key for each form, e.g. for differing male and female organisms, or for the different stages in the life cycle of insects. Although it may happen that the specimens are collected from a large population so that different forms of what are presumably the same taxon can be found in association, the key writer cannot assume that all the alternative forms are available and must not use characters from different forms in the same key.

Finally, a key must be tested after it has been constructed. The usual way to do this is to try it out with an adequate selection of correctly identified additional specimens, other than those used in the compilation. It is best for some person other than the author to do this to avoid bias. Errors which may be encountered are errors of fact (in the data matrix), or errors made in the actual construction of the key. It may also happen that the characters are not weighted as sensibly as they might be, or that commonly occurring variations in the taxa have not been allowed for. It may not be wise to alter the key in order to allow for every observed variation or aberration since, if these are included, the essential distinctions between taxa may be obscured or destroyed. The writing of a key often proceeds along with the revision of a taxonomic group, and if descriptions of taxa are also being written, these must agree exactly with the key. Some authors put facts in the key which are not repeated in the corresponding descriptive text, so that information has to be sought in several places. This practice is not recommended.

4.1.3 Other forms

The two previous sections described common forms of the diagnostic key, but other varieties exist. So far, questions have been distinguished by numbering them, but some authors prefer to use letters. For longer keys this requires the use of repeated letters, e.g. 'AA', or of other alphabets, and the result can be untidy.

In order to save space on the printed page, one can abandon the use of a new line for every fresh lead, and use a prominent typeface, e.g. '**bold**', for the question numbers and taxon names, so that it is still possible to trace a path through the compressed text of the key. A 'solid' key in this form is not very attractive. Keys with drawings incorporated into the leads are very presentable, but perhaps more expensive to publish. An example is given in Fig. 4.1 (Chinery, 1973). Such keys are most helpful for beginners and for teaching purposes. The choice of an organism to illustrate presents some difficulties, especially at the higher levels, because, however typical the illustration, actual specimens are likely to differ considerably from it at times.

A more special form of key is one where contrasting leads of the same question are given different, instead of the same, numbers. The number of the next contrasting lead is given in brackets. Leads, starting from the first are labelled 1a, 1b, etc., until a taxon is keyed out, when the lead number is changed to 2, and so on. This results in a key which also indexes the taxa by the lead numbers. It does not seem to have become widely popular.

Synoptic keys are sometimes published, which look just like conventional keys, but are keys intended to present a classification, rather than to identify actual taxa. The classification may well have been simplified or idealised, so such a key should not be used to make identifications.

Yet another type of key exists which begins to look more like a tabular key (p. 105), but its total effect is actually just like that of a diagnostic key, since all specimens must necessarily agree with all the characters used. Rypka (1971) calls it a *truth table*. An example is given in Fig. 4.2, which is based on the *Epilobium* data of Fig. 1.1 A certain number of good characters are chosen to

Key to the Orders of European Insects

1. Insects winged   2
   Insects wingless or with vestigial wings   28

2. One pair of wings   3
   Two pairs of wings   7

3. Body grasshopper-like, with enlarged   Orthoptera
   hind legs and pronotum extending
   back over abdomen

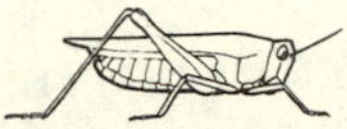

   Insect not like this   4

4. Abdomen with 'tails'   5
   Abdomen without 'tails'   6

5. Insects <5mm long, with relatively   Hemiptera
   long antennae: wing with only one
   forked vein

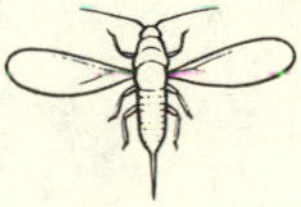

   Larger insects with short   Ephemeroptera
   antennae and many wing
   veins: tails relatively long

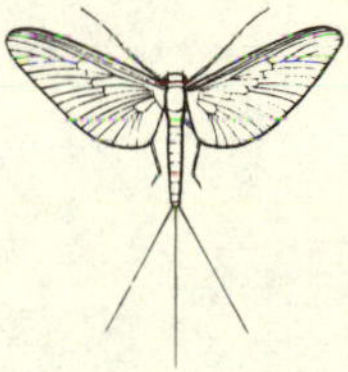

6. Front wings forming club-shaped   Strepsiptera
   halteres

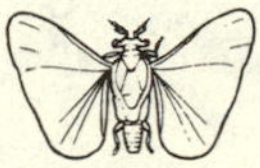

   Hind wings forming halteres   Diptera
   (may be hidden)

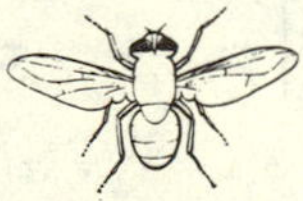

7. Front wings hard or leathery   8
   All wings membranous   13

8. Front wings horny except for   Hemiptera
   membranous tip

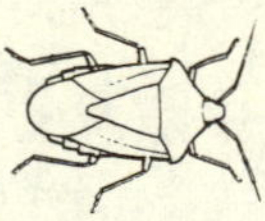

   Front wings of uniform texture throughout   9

Fig. 4.1 Example of illustrated key (after Chinery).

A ALL TAXA

Truth value	Character no.			Taxa
	4	5	10	
0	0	0	0	10
1	0	0	1	3
2	0	1	0	Group 1
3	0	1	1	Group 2
4	1	0	0	1
5	1	0	1	2
6	1	1	0	5
7	1	1	1	6

Character 4　no – 0
　　　　　yes – 1
5　terete – 0
　lined – 1
10　cuneate – 0
　　rounded – 1

B TAXA GROUP 1

Truth value	Character no.		Taxa
	7	13	
0	0	0	(5,6,10,13)
1	0	1	4
2	0	2	8
3	1	0	11
4	1	1	7
5	1	2	(1)

Character 7　no – 0
　　　　　yes – 1
Character 13　< 6mm – 0
　　　　　6–10mm – 1
　　　　　>10mm – 2

C TAXA GROUP 2

Truth value	Character 1	Taxa
0	0	9
1	1	12
2	2	13

Character 1:　erect – 0
　　　　　decumbent – 1
　　　　　prostrate – 2

Fig. 4.2 Truth table for British species of *Epilobium*.

begin the key, in Table A. In this case there are three, each with two states, making in all $2^3 = 8$ possible combinations of states. The states are numbered 0 and 1, and when the combinations are written out they become the same as binary numbers (as used in digital computers). For example, the combination 101, regarded as a binary number, is the same as the decimal number 5. This is called the *truth value*, and acts as an index number for the various combinations. In order to identify a specimen one must establish the character state combination which applies, and look for the taxon numbers given at the right. If there is just one taxon, as number 2 for value 5, then the identification is complete. If there is no taxon, as in rows 0 and 5 of Table B, then there must be an error. The taxon numbers given in brackets in Table B really belong in other tables. If there are several taxa, as in rows 2 and 3 of Table A, additional tables are required to separate them (B and C). There is no compulsion to use only binary characters as, for example, Table B includes character 13 which has 3 states. It is not essential to number states from zero, or to use numbers at all. Some keys have letter codes for the states instead. A key of this type is best suited for situations where characters are best evaluated in groups, or as batches of tests.

4.1.4 Theory

The most useful results are set out here with a minimum of mathematics, and without proof. For more details see Osborne (1963).

Firstly, there is a fixed relation between the number of taxa (T) and the number of questions (Q) in a dichotomous key, namely

$$Q=T-1$$

In the keys of Figs. 1.4 and 1.5 the number of questions Q is 12, and the number of taxa T is 13, which illustrates this theorem. Although the number of ways to construct a key for a given set of taxa is very large, the number of questions required will always be the same. If a key is not strictly dichotomous, i.e. some questions contain more than two leads, then Q may be reduced, and the theorem is no longer exact. If taxa are variable, and have to be keyed out in more than one place in a key, then T represents the effective number of taxa including these additions.

There is a connection between the number of taxa which key out at various levels of a key, and the numbers of the levels. For example, the key in Fig. 1.3 has six levels, and the number of taxa t, which key out at level i are

i	1	2	3	4	5	6
t_i	1	0	0	5	5	2

The total number of levels (L) is 6
The relation is

$$\sum_{i=1}^{L} 2^{-i}\, t_i = 1$$

In this example the left hand side is

$$\frac{1.1}{2} + \frac{0.1}{4} + \frac{0.1}{8} + \frac{5.1}{16} + \frac{5.1}{32} + \frac{2.1}{64}$$

which adds up to 1.

The theory of errors in keys is generally rather complex (Osborne, 1963), but the following simple argument is quite illuminating. Assume that the probability that each question is answered correctly is p, and that all questions are equally likely to be answered correctly. Then the probability that both the first questions will be answered correctly is p^2, and so for a key with L levels, the probability of getting a correct identification is approximately p^L, because the number of questions to be answered before identifying a taxon is, on average, about the same as the number of levels. Suppose $p = 0.9$, i.e. there is a 90% chance of answering each question correctly (or a 10% chance of getting it wrong). With $L = 6$, as in the example key (Figs. 1.3-1.5), $p^L = (0.9)^6$, which is roughly 0.5. In other words, even with such a short key as this, the chances of getting a right answer are only even, or 50%! In reality p is not the same for all questions, and must be a good deal better than 90% if keys are going to work. Also, the actual value of p will not be known, but instead one may only know that some characters are more reliable than others. If an error occurs in using a key, and a question is answered wrongly, the wrong lead is followed, and the key user continues in the wrong part of the key. The nearer the beginning of the key this happens, the worse the consequences may be. Hence, other things being equal, reliable characters are best used first in the key, and the less reliable ones later, so as to lessen the consequences of possible errors.

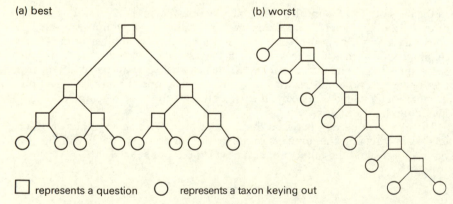

(a) best   (b) worst

☐ represents a question   ◯ represents a taxon keying out

Fig. 4.3   Tree diagrams for the best and worst cases of average path length in keys for 8 taxa.

It is also clear that a key will be more reliable if the average path length for the taxa, which is the average number of questions to be answered in order to key out a specimen, is as small as possible. Two extreme cases are shown in

Fig. 4.3. The average path length in case (a) is 3, and for case (b) is

$$\frac{1}{8} \ (1+2+3+4+5+6+7+7) \ = \ 4\frac{3}{8}$$

Intuitively one can see that the 'best' key of case (a) is arrived at by constructing the key so that at each question the taxa are divided equally into each lead. It may not be possible to do this exactly, owing to the way in which the states of actual characters are distributed, and the number of taxa will not usually be a power of 2 as it was in the above example. Hence one may say that a better key is likely to be produced if each question divides the taxa into two sets which are as equal as possible, and that this policy tends to give the shortest average path length. This is not always the case, however, because counter examples can be constructed. This is, therefore, not a mathematical theorem but a useful rule of thumb.

There is a relation between the minimum number of levels L and the number of taxa T. This can be seen in the idealised key, case (a) in Fig. 4.3 If there are two taxa, one question will be enough to separate them. For four, three questions will be needed, one at level one and two at level two. In the example, 8 taxa are keyed out in 3 levels. One can see that, by continuing this process, L levels can take at most 2^L taxa, so

$$2^L = T$$
$$\text{or, } L = \log_2 T$$

Obviously, this is the extreme case, so in general

$$L > = \log_2 T$$

4.1.5 Multi-access keys on punched cards

These occur in two distinct forms, the *edge-punched* key, (Fig. 4.4) and the *body-punched* key or *feature card* (Fig. 4.5).

In an edge-punched key, there is one card to each taxon. The states of characters are represented by holes around the margin, and the area of the card may be ruled off so that character state names can be written in, or else these can be specially printed in advance, as shown in Fig. 4.4, which was designed by Whalley. If a taxon shows a certain character state, the corresponding hole is clipped out, e.g. for 'eyes smooth', number 17 in Fig. 4.4. Conversely, one could choose to punch out a hole if the character does not occur. In order to use the key, the cards are sorted by a needle. Suppose a specimen has 'eyes smooth', then the needle is pushed through hole 17, and the pack of cards is shaken, then all cards for all taxa which agree with this will fall out. All cards which disagree (i.e. those for 'eyes hairy', the converse) remain in the pack. At this stage, it is possible to choose a good character, in the sense of a character which is more effective at eliminating taxa, by looking at the edge of the pack of cards for unused characters. A good character will have about half the holes punched out, if it is a two-state character. Another character is chosen, and the sorting repeated, until just one card remains, corresponding to the identified taxon.

This kind of key is strictly monothetic, since only one character can be

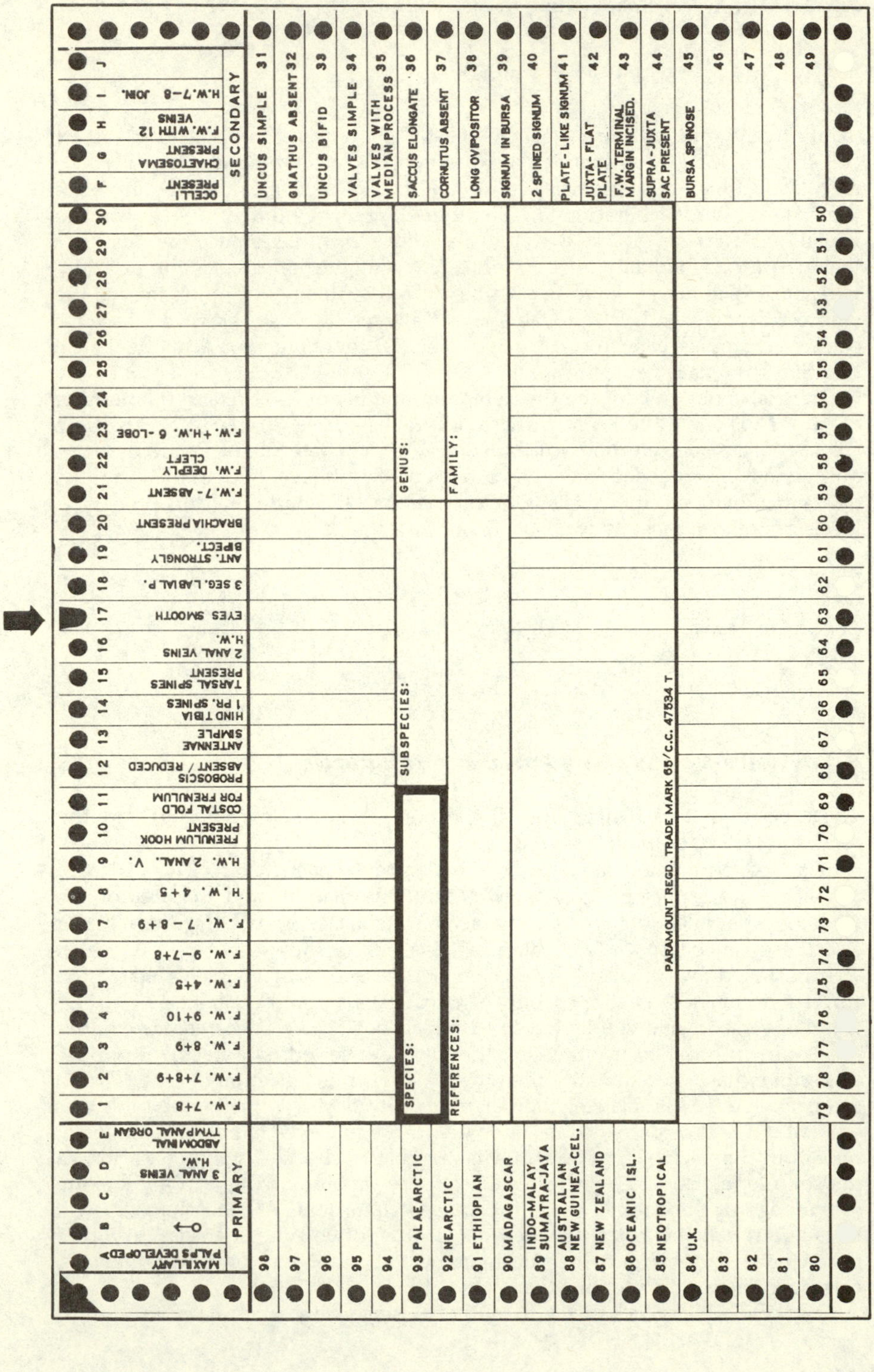

Fig. 4.4 Edge-punched card from key to *Lepidoptera*.

used at a time. The number of characters which can be covered is restricted by the perimeter of the card, and about 100 character states are possible in Fig. 4.4. The number of taxa which can be included is not limited, except by convenience. There is no need to keep the cards in any particular order. In the example quoted, no allowance has been made for variable or missing characters. If there was a taxon which could have either 'eyes smooth' or 'eyes hairy', then the key as described could go wrong, unless separate holes were punched for both 'eyes smooth' and 'eyes hairy'. On the other hand conditional characters, e.g. 'wing shape' for a wingless insect, must not be punched at all because with actual specimens, one would never try to use such a character! It is not easy to reproduce mechanically copies of keys of this kind, and they tend to be made in very small numbers. The identification of a taxon made with this kind of key can be easily confirmed by looking at the other holes on the margin of the remaining card. If a wrong identification is suspected, the key cannot easily be worked backwards, and it is better to start again.

Body-punched keys differ in that holes are punched in rows and columns over the area of the card, and not just on its edge. Each card represents a character state printed on it, e.g. 'milky juice present' in Fig. 4.5 (taken from Hansen and Rahn, 1969). The holes, which are identified by a number found by looking at column and row numbers on the card, each represent one taxon. If a hole is punched out, this means that the taxon concerned shows, or could show, the character in that state. For example, the hole number 320 in Fig. 4.5 shows that the family Compositae has character state number 6. There

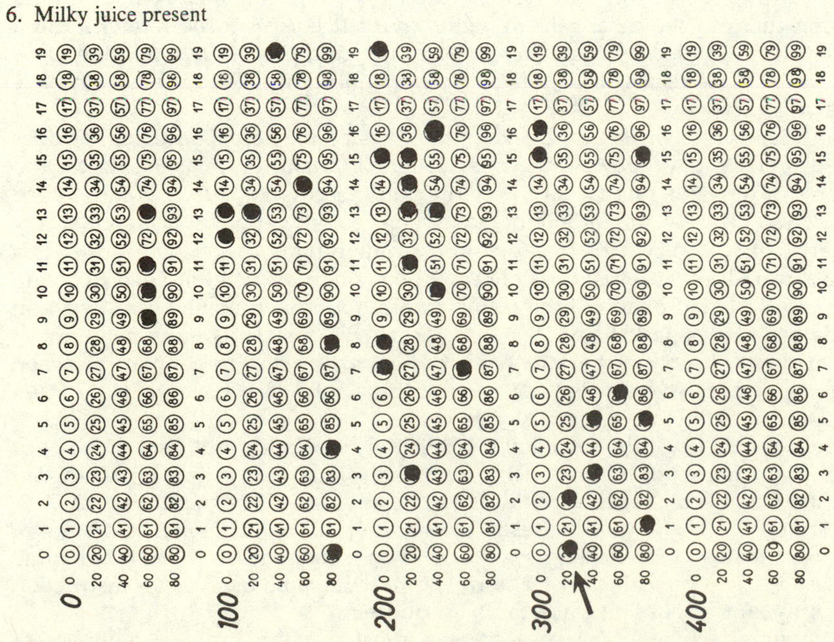

6. Milky juice present

Fig. 4.5 Card from key to angiosperm families (after Hansen and Rahn).

is a separate list of numbers for taxa (families in this case). The key is used by taking out the cards for character states shown by the specimen, and overlapping them precisely. Any taxa which agree with all the character states will show a hole right through when the cards are held up to the light, or laid on a dark background. When only one hole shows, then look up the number of the hole to find the name of the taxon which has been identified.

This key is more or less monothetic, but there is the possibility that if a hole is only blocked by one or two cards, this will still be visible, so that taxa which do not quite agree can still be recognised. This depends on the thickness and nature of the material from which the cards are made. If semitransparent, coloured or grey plastic is used for such a key, it could permit taxa to be identified correctly even when there are errors, provided the material is neither too pale nor too dark. Any number of characters can be used, but the number of taxa is restricted by the area of the card. In the example (Fig. 4.5) this is 500 and is not really prohibitive. It is convenient to keep the cards in a fixed sequence so that characters can be found when wanted, but after an identification has been carried out the cards have to be put back in the right place. Sometimes cards are pinned together at a corner and rotated in a fan in order to overlay them, but it can then be difficult to get them properly in line unless there is only quite a small number of them. Variable characters are dealt with by punching a hole in each card which corresponds to a possible state. As before, inapplicable characters must be left out of the key completely. Body-punched keys are more readily reproduced in quantity than edge-punched cards, but still require special equipment, unless computer cards are used (but see p. 139). The identification of a taxon can be confirmed by pulling out further cards for supplementary characters and adding them to the cards already withdrawn. It is easy to back-track from a wrong identification by removing some of the cards previously selected. This is especially useful when there is no hole common to all the cards which have been withdrawn!

Both kinds of punched card key operate by step-by-step elimination, as does the diagnostic key. However, any selection of characters may be used, and in any order, and this is why they are multi-access keys (sometimes called *polyclaves*). This is an important advantage for incomplete or fragmentary material. It is also possible to stop short of identifying a specimen down to a single taxon if the material does not provide enough information, and to obtain a short list of taxon names for a result. In other words, punched card keys can easily be used as partial keys. They are, however, just as likely to fail if errors are made in observing characters as are diagnostic keys. In general, punched card keys are not very convenient to publish, and hence have not very often been encountered in the past.

Multi-access keys are sometimes published by writing out lists of taxa for each character state, without using punched cards. For example, using Fig. 1.1, the taxa which have, or could have, 'leaves sessile' are numbers 1, 2, 7, 9, 10, 11 and 13. The key is then used by working through a sequence of chosen character states, and rejecting any taxon whose number does not occur in all the lists. A key published in this form can of course be used as an instruction kit for making a set of punched cards for oneself.

Although punched card keys are the most popular form of multi-access key, mechanical equivalents also exist. An instance of this is the 'information sorter' (Olds, 1970) which uses transparent plastic sheets instead of cards, one for each character, mounted in a cabinet with internal lighting. The sheets are ruled in three squares for each taxon (microbes), mounted behind a plate with square holes in it, and they can slide to a left, right or central position, corresponding to 'absent', 'present' or 'not used'. The holes in the plate correspond to the central square on the slide when the slide is in its central position. The squares are tinted red for character states which do not agree with a taxon and a green filter is usually switched in to make a contrast. There is a button for sliding the sheet for each character into place, and taxa which agree show as a green square on the front of the machine.

4.2 Identification by comparison

The method of comparison, or matching, is straightforward in principle. The unknown specimen is first examined and its characters are observed or investigated by experiment. It is then compared with all of the taxa of an appropriate group and identified with whichever of these agrees exactly, or is the most similar. The comparison of the specimen with the reference taxa may involve counting the number of characters which agree, or calculating some measure of the agreement (a similarity coefficient) based on character matches and mismatches. The result of the comparison may also be a short list of taxa rather than just one, from which a subjective choice must be made.

The simplest form of this method is that of direct comparison, where one takes the specimen and looks through a book of illustrations, or photographs, or through a collection of preserved specimens, until one finds a taxon which 'looks the same'. No objective assessment of similarity or identity may be used at all, or at any rate, not consciously. This is what many people would naturally do to identify or 'name' something, in the sense described on p. 1; they take a popular handbook on natural history, e.g. on birds, and just thumb through the pages in order to 'find a picture of it'. However, it may be difficult to make this visual assessment without considerable practice if the taxa are numerous and very much alike. Also, if there are no reference collections or illustrations, but only a flora, handbook or monograph with purely written descriptions, the comparisons are much harder to make without some visual aid.

Comparison methods have the advantage that they do not demand any particular characters from the specimen and can be used successfully with incomplete material. The characters are used all together, polythetically and as the outcome does not depend on the correct observation of every character, some errors can be tolerated. However, the results become more reliable as more characters are used, and so a detailed and perhaps tedious examination of the specimen may be called for. Also, if there are many taxa to consider, there may be much labour involved in comparing the specimen with every taxon.

4.2.1 Tabular methods

These may take a variety of different forms, but the basic procedure can be illustrated from Fig. 1.1 for *Epilobium*. The figure shows a rectangular table giving the data matrix for this genus. Species are in columns, and characters

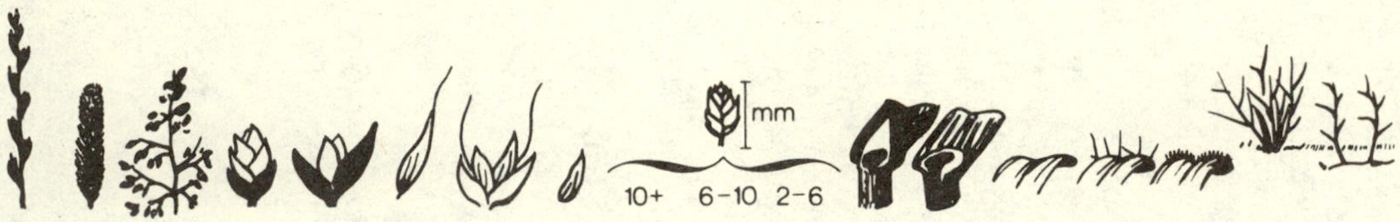

False Brome *(Brachypodium sylvaticum)*
Italian Ryegrass *(Lolium multiflorum)*
Perennial Ryegrass *(L. perenne)*
Common Couch *(Agropyron repens)*
Bearded Couch *(A. caninum)*
Crested Dogstail *(Cynosurus cristatus)*
Wall Barley *(Hordeum murinum)*
Sweet Vernal-grass *(Anthoxanthum odoratum)*
Meadow Foxtail *(Alopecurus pratensis)*
Timothy *(Phleum pratense)*
Yorkshire-fog *(Holcus lanatus)*
Creeping Softgrass *(H. mollis)*
Tufted Hairgrass *(Deschcmpsia cespitosa)*

mm   10+   6–10   2–6

■ YES   ◉ USUALLY NO   ○ NO   ✱ INAPPLICABLE

Fig. 4.6   Part of lateral key to common British grasses (after Sinker).

in rows. The entries in the table are the states of the characters in abbreviated form, e.g. by character 1, 'stem habit', E stands for 'erect'. A new specimen of *Epilobium* is examined and each of the available characters is written down the edge of a sheet of paper, using the same abbreviations as in the table. Move the paper across the table, column by column, noting the number of disagreements for each. If only one species is found which entirely agrees, that will be the identification; otherwise, one could take the species with the fewest disagreements as the answer. If there are several which disagree to the same extent, a choice between them will have to be made in some other way, e.g. by comparing with a collection of preserved specimens. Notice that the disagreements were counted, not the agreements. This is because the number of characters available for comparison varies from species to species because of missing or conditional characters. Alternatively, the proportion of agreements could be used, instead of the total, but this extra calculation for each taxon becomes a little tedious to carry out with pencil and paper.

Another variety of the tabular key appears in Hedge and Lamond (1972) and in Tutin (1980), both applied to the plant family Umbelliferae. Here the states of 9 characters are represented by capital letters, and the user is invited to describe his specimen and write down the 9 appropriate letters in a formula which is then used to look up the correct combination in a table. This table is in alphabetical order, and may lead to the name of a species or to a subsidiary diagnostic key for a genus. If any of the requested characters are missing from the specimen then the partial formula may match several entries in the table, each of which must then be explored further. As it stands, this type of key is limited to 26 character states, but it could be extended by using other symbols, e.g. Greek alphabet, or numerical formulae with one digit for each character, when it becomes a truth table. When the formulae get long and there are more missing characters, the method becomes tedious.

An improvement on the tabular method is the *lateral key* (Fig. 4.6) devised by Sinker (1975). There is a column for every state of every character, not just for each character as in Fig. 1.1 The characters are marked off by vertical lines. Each position in the table is filled with a symbol. The user is provided with, or can make for himself, a strip of card with tabs which can be folded over. The tabs are the same width as the columns. The specimen is examined, and the tabs are folded back for each character state observed. The strip is then slid down the table. The taxon which is the correct one will display only black squares (for 'yes') and perhaps some of the signs for 'variable' when the strip is covering the right row of the table. The other symbols, for 'no' and 'inapplicable' will remain covered by tabs which have not been turned down. The advantage of this version is that it is easy to assess visually whether the specimen agrees with a taxon without needing to count the number of agreements.

4.2.2 Mechanical methods

Mechanical equivalents of tables have also been tried. One version consists of a transparent plastic slide on which the description of the specimen is written (Cowan and Steel, 1960). Underneath this a board is placed on which the table has been drawn. The slide is moved over the table until a row of the table beneath is seen to agree. An improved version of this has been called the 'logoscope' (Nash, 1960) and resembles a slide rule (Fig. 4.7). The table of data is divided into strips, one for each character (symptom or sign), and the user picks out only those strips for the characters which he wishes to use. The strips are marked with a line for a taxon (disease) if the character is present, and left blank otherwise. The strips are put into the bed of the device,

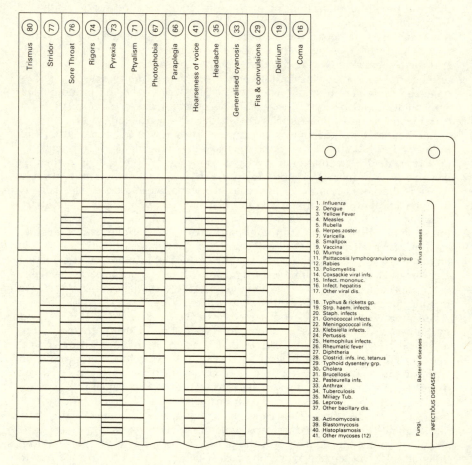

Fig. 4.7 The logoscope; example for diagnosis of rabies (disease 12) (after Nash).

and a slide can be moved over them to help detect a continuous or nearly continuous line, representing agreement or partial agreement with a taxon. The user is recommended to use as many characters as possible. This device could be used either as a multi-access key, using step-by-step elimination (as in a body-punched card key), or else as a tabular identification method. Some errors in character observation can be tolerated, since they give rise to a nearly complete line across the bed of the device and this is easily seen.

4.3 Mixed methods

The distinction between an elimination method and a matching method is not hard and fast. When discussing the use of a diagnostic key with the *Epilobium* example (p. 89), there was the possibility that a lead might have several characters, and that neither side of the couplet might agree exactly. The sensible action to take in such circumstances is to choose the alternative which agrees best, or has the highest score. The user of the key is really making a mental estimate of a similarity coefficient. The key by Gauld (1980) to genera of *Ophion* goes further, and at certain leads, requires the user to record a group of characters, calculate a score, and then continue with one of two new leads according to whether the score is above or below a threshold value.

5

Computerised identification methods

The methods which may or must involve computations are discussed here. The calculations are often somewhat lengthy or complex, so that the use of a computer is usual although not essential. Desktop or pocket calculators, or pencil and paper could also be used. Some of the methods involve the computer indirectly (diagnostic and punched card keys), while others use it directly (matching and on-line). The related problem of character set minimisation is discussed, as well as techniques requiring special equipment other than computers. Finally, a critical comparison of the methods is made, so that one can see how to choose a method appropriate to a particular problem.

5.1 Data format

Before a computer can make use of taxonomic data for identification, the data must be coded or represented in some way; this is called the data format. The data to be represented include the descriptions of the characters in terms of the states which occur, and the names of the taxa, together with other details such as character and taxon weights if required.

The way in which the data are represented is essentially a compromise between what is convenient for human beings, and what is convenient for computation. To humans, descriptions of taxa are most easily understood as pictures, and also in writing. Computers manipulate facts most readily if they are in numerical form, because in this form programs are easier to write and the machines run faster. While it is possible to have computers read descriptions of taxa in the form in which they usually appear in textbooks, i.e. as a simplified form of ordinary language, it is cheaper and more convenient to code the facts as numbers, to some extent at least.

The example of a data format discussed below is not necessarily claimed to be the ultimate and ideal format. Other formats could be designed to impart the same information more or less effeciently, and a discussion of the principles of data format design follows. In general, two types of format are frequently encountered, fixed and free. Fixed format means that numbers and words are expected to occur in a regular sequence. For example, a common form of input used to be the 80-column punched card, and it was customary to punch numbers on these with equal spacing, e.g. one to every space of five columns, and in such a way that each number was right-adjusted, i.e. placed at the right-hand end of its space. In fixed format, any number which is not in its correct place may be misread. With free format, on the other hand, the items of data need only to be separated by spaces or some other punctuation mark and can be spread out as desired, without regard to the position on a line. Fixed format input is often used with the FORTRAN programming language, commonly used for scientific purposes. Free format is more convenient for the user, but takes a little more programming.

The data format which is used in the following discussion is known as DELTA (short for DEscription Language for TAxonomy) and was invented by Dallwitz (1980). When the first edition of this book was written, there were a variety of data formats in use, but in the meantime DELTA has become an international standard, and its use is strongly recommended. Taxonomic programs which are not based on a standard format can have only rather limited applications. DELTA is a *free* format. This represents an improvement over the older *fixed* formats, where the data had to be set out in a rigid manner. This means that the computer now has an extra program for interpreting the data correctly, and that the effort has shifted away from the user and towards the machine.

DELTA files contain two kinds of information, directives and data. Directives serve to give parameters of the file, such as the number of species, and divide up the data into sections. They are often self-explanatory. They all begin with an asterisk, e.g.

*NUMBER OF CHARACTERS 34

The example given below is based on data for moths *(Lepidoptera)*. For ease of understanding, we shall first consider the definition of characters and states, which follows the directive

*CHARACTER LIST

Characters are numbered in sequence starting from one, and the states which apply to them are also numbered, separately for each character. The clear distinction between the concept of the character, and the states which apply to it, is vital to the subsequent processing of the descriptions. Hence the character 'Presence of proboscis' with two states 'absent' and 'present' could appear as

#1. Proboscis <presence>/
  1. absent/
  2. present/

The numero sign (#) marks the beginning of a new character, the slash (/) shows where a string of characters ends, and the angle brackets (<>) enclose a comment. Either upper or lower case letters are allowed. The definition just given does more than give 'absent' and 'present' as the states of the character, since it also means that these are the only states which can apply to it. The character was defined as 'Proboscis <presence>' so that the character string can be combined with either of the state strings to make a readable phrase for use in descriptions and keys, e.g. 'Proboscis present'. The word 'presence' is a comment which is ignored for such purposes. If there are other characters of the proboscis, e.g. 'Proboscis <length>', then the comment may be retained whenever a list of the characters is needed, so that different characters of the proboscis can be distinguished. The first character could also have been defined as 'Proboscis presence', without the comment marks, but this would permit ugly phrasing, such as 'Proboscis presence present'. Some characters may be a little more awkward to express, such as 'male' versus 'female'. The character could be called 'Gender', but it is not usual to write 'Gender male', since 'male' on its own is enough. In this situation, all that is needed is a comment, and the character name can be left out, e.g.

> #5. <Gender>/
> > 1. Male/
> > 2. Female/

Characters can in fact have any number of states, and not just two as in the above examples.

So far, the examples have only been for qualitative characters. Suppose that we wish to have a character for 'Length of wing', which varies in practice from 5 to 20 mm. This could be approximated as a qualitative character, e.g.

> #10. Wing <length>/
> > 1. up to 10mm/
> > 2. 10 to 15mm/
> > 3. over 15mm/

This will prove awkward if a description happens to just overlap two of these artificial states. A taxon with wings 8-12mm long would have to go in both states 1 and 2, and would then effectively have a wing length of 0-15mm, which is a distortion of the facts. A better approximation could be made by increasing the number of states, e.g. 'up to 6mm', '6-8mm', '8-10mm' etc., but this is awkward when the actual descriptions are coded (see below). The easiest way is to define 'Wing length' directly as a continuously variable (real) character;

> #10. Wing <length>/ mm/

and to give the actual range of measurements in the subsequent descriptions. In this example there is an extra (optional) string 'mm' for the units. No strings for the character states are needed, as there are none. Discrete (integer) variables are defined in a similar way, e.g.

> #11. Setae on 2nd segment <number>/

In spite of what has just been said, there is sometimes a need to express a quantitative character as separate states (a *pseudoqualitative* character), and it is possible to do this with a special directive, KEY STATES, which is described below. This allows the actual measurements to be given in the descriptions, and leaves the computer to create the qualitative states when required.

The ideal way to describe a quantitative character would be to state its statistical distribution with parameters, e.g. normal, with mean and standard deviation. However, the labour required to establish this kind of data for biological identification usually makes it impractical, and measurements are usually quoted as a range, e.g. '5-15 cm', or less often as '(2) 5-15 (20) cm', meaning that the extremes (2-5, or 15-20 cm) are less often encountered. This could be given a little more precision by recording the frequency of different measurements, and giving the ends of the range as percentiles, say at 10% and 90%. This would mean that 20% of specimens measure less than 5 or more than 15 cm. The simplest solution is to denote the ends of the range and the unit of measurement, if any.

Now that characters have been defined, one can set out the descriptions of taxa. This is done after the directive

*ITEM DESCRIPTIONS

Each taxon begins with an item which gives its name, e.g.

#1. Banisia furva/

which is followed by the description on subsequent lines. Each character with its state or states is represented by a character number and the state number(s), e.g.

1,2   means   'Proboscis present'

Similarly

11,3   means   'No. of setae is 3'

and

10,5-8   means   'Wing is 5 to 8 mm long'

Variation is permitted in every kind of character, so

1,1<rarely>/2 means   'Proboscis absent or present'

where 'rarely' is a comment, and

11,3/5/7-9

means that the number of setae is 3, 5 or 7 to 9. If a character is completely variable, this can be written as 'V', e.g.

1,V means the same as 1,1/2

There is a particular kind of variation which causes difficulty, which is when two character states occur together, which could be expressed as 'and' or 'with'. As an example of this situation, consider the description of forewing venation in a family of moths. The veins are numbered, and '+' means, roughly speaking, 'joined to'. There could be six different situations, expressible in the data as:

#3. Forewing veins <branching>/
    1. 7+8/
    2. 7+8+9 <two kinds>/
    3. 8+9+10/
    4. 8+9/
    5. 9+10/
    6. 7+8 with 9+10/

Comments are allowed in states also, as in number 2. The DELTA format allows descriptions to be written as

3,1&5   meaning   '7+8' and '9+10'

This is no problem if the data is only to be used for printing descriptions, but if the data is to be used for identification purposes, then this is inadmissible. This is because a wing with 7+8 venation is different from a wing with 9+10 venation which is different again from a wing which has both. Hence 1&5 is really a new state, distinct from 1 and from 5, and the additional state 6 should be used to express it.

For programming purposes, it is often convenient to actually store variable characters as a sum of numbers from the sequence 1, 2, 4, 8 etc., representing each state 1, 2, 3, 4 etc. This allows every possible variation to be represented uniquely. This would not be a very convenient way to record the data in the format, but it is a suitable way to store and process variable characters in the computer. This is because digital computer arithmetic is mostly based on the number 2, rather than the more familiar arithmetic of decimal numbers (base 10). It then becomes a simple matter to test by computer whether a taxon shows a particular state of a variable character or not, and to decide whether two taxa with various states of a given character are distinct or not.

There are two special situations where states of characters are unknown (missing) or inapplicable. There is an important difference between these two situations. If a character is unknown, more research or fieldwork can be undertaken to discover it. If a character is inapplicable, its occurrence is logically impossible. In the format, unknown is expressed as 'U', and inapplicable as '-'. To illustrate this, consider character 3 above (vein branching). If this pattern is '7 + 8 + 9' (state 2), there are two possibilities, expressed in character 4, viz:

> #4.   Forewings <7 + 8 + 9>/
> 1. 9 from 7 + 8/
> 2. 7 from 8 + 9/

So for a taxon with veins 7 to 9 joined in the second way, character 3 = 2 and character 4 = 2. If character 3 had state 2, but character 4 had just been overlooked, then character 4 = U. If however, character 3 has state 1 (veins 7 and 8 joined, but not 9), then character 4 = -, because it means nothing. If character 3 = 3 and 4 = 1, this would mean venation could be '7 + 8' or '7 + 8 + 9', and if and only if the latter, it is '9 from 7 + 8'.

In order to distinguish between missing and inapplicable characters, the computer will need to know that there is a condition that says 'you cannot have character 4 if character 3 = 1, etc.', and this will also have to be put in the data. These rules are placed under the directive

> *DEPENDENT CHARACTERS 3,1:4

which means 'if 3 equals 1 you can't have 4'.

We now return to the directives at the beginning of the format. The first to appear is the heading, e.g.

> *HEADING   Moths of genus Banisia/

There are several directives for stating the number of taxa and the number of characters, e.g.

> *MAXIMUM NUMBER OF ITEMS 34
> *NUMBER OF CHARACTERS 15

Characters can have different types, e.g.

> *CHARACTER TYPES 3,OM 10,RN 14,IN 23,TE

This states that character 10 is a real number, 14 is an integer, and that 3 is an ordered multistate. The reason for this is that the states of some characters have an ascending or descending order, e.g. sizes, and this can affect the way that descriptions are written. Lastly, 23 is a text character, which has no states but is just used as a comment.

Multistate qualitative characters can have different numbers of states, and these are given in the directive

    *NUMBERS OF STATES 3,6

Weights for characters and for taxa, if required, can appear in the directives

    *CHARACTER WEIGHTS

and

    *ITEM WEIGHTS

as a list of pairs of numbers; the number of the character or taxon and the weight itself. Characters may be weighted in such a way that the weights are actually used in the computations, e.g. one might state that one character was 10 times better than another, or else just signify the order in which characters are to be used. The weights of taxa usually signify the frequencies in which they are expected to occur.

As mentioned above, there are times when quantitative characters need to be expressed in qualitative terms as well. For this, the directive

    *KEY STATES   10,0-5/5-10/10-20

is used, for example. This splits the character 10 into three ranges, as in the earlier example, but has the advantage that the actual measurements can be stored in the descriptions, and do not need to be recoded when the user wants to change the divisions. It is possible to let the ranges overlap, e.g.

    *KEY STATES   10,0-6/4-11/9-20

but this is not recommended, because it leads to non-exclusive character states. Care is needed even when the ranges are contiguous, since with the ranges set, for example, at 0-5/5-10, a value of 5 could be assigned to both 0-5 and 5-10, i.e. equivalent to 0-10, which is a distortion. This problem can be avoided by expressing the ranges more precisely, e.g.

    *KEY STATES   10,0-4.9/5-9.9/10-20

These difficulties are part of a general problem, which recurs elsewhere, of the effects of mixing range data with single values in quantitative characters. It may seem convenient to score, for example, 'wings 5mm' but this does not mix well with another score like 'wings 4-8mm'. It is recommended that observations of real variables are always made with a range of variation. A statement like 'wings 5mm' is not strictly accurate in any case; it is unlikely that wings of all specimens are exactly and only 5mm long.

Once the data have been completely scored, the computer can help to check for correctness. If fixed format is used, this will first mean that all items which have a fixed position must occur where they are expected. A data format such as that outlined above has a certain amount of redundant information in it. This is done deliberately in order to assist checking. For example, one could manage without numbering the characters and their states, provided that one was certain that they were in the correct order. The computer can check that this is so if the characters and states are numbered. The number of states for each character is given, and hence the maximum possible score for each character can be found. For a binary character this is $1 + 2 = 3$, for a 3-state character it is $1 + 2 + 4 = 7$, and in general for an m-state character, it is $(2^m - 1)$. Any entry in the matrix which is greater than this is clearly wrong. Similarly, the code for inapplicable (-1) should only occur if the character concerned is known to depend on another character, and if that controlling character has the appropriate state(s).

Apart from making the data self-consistent, there are other ways in which it can be refined. It is usual practice only to include characters which vary within the group of taxa concerned. The computer can check that this is in fact so, and if not, state which of the characters are redundant. One can then make alterations so that the characters are no longer redundant, or they can be weighted so that they are ignored, or they can be taken out altogether. Usually all of the taxa are supposed to be different from each other. The computer can compare all of them with one another in pairs, and report on any pairs which are not distinct. It often happens that two taxa are not identical, but have no characters whose states do not overlap, which is what is meant by 'not distinct'. The cure is to redefine the taxa slightly or add new and diagnostic characters. On the other hand, one may wish to continue and produce partial keys instead of complete ones and be content if some taxa cannot be separated.

Once the data is syntactically correct, according to the rules of the format, there is still the problem of making sure that it is correct factually. The situation here is no different from other areas of data processing, and the only way to check it is to proof read it, and this is best done by another person. The description printing programs can be a great help here, since the numerical part of the format is converted to words. DELTA descriptive data is in taxon order, but it may sometimes be convenient to view it in character order instead, and to list which taxa possess particular character states. This can be done interactively with one of the online identification programs. The result of this operation is in effect the same as writing a lateral or synoptic key, which is just the data matrix written out in a different way. Several authors (Rhoades, 1986 and Anderegg, 1989) have written programs specifically in order to do this, in conjunction with an online identification program (not based on DELTA however).

The DELTA format has been presented without reference to any database systems, since historically it was designed some years before suitable systems became available. DELTA is also more complex in its data structures than many database systems will allow. However, there is no doubt that in due course, DELTA will be converted into a database in the proper sense. There are already data capture programs which can assist with the collection and editing of descriptive data. The first of these was described in the context of writing floras by computer (Pankhurst, 1983b). The questionnaire program (COND4) is driven by a DELTA definition of characters and states, and will present a menu for each character in turn, prompting the user to type in states for the current character. The program takes character dependency into account, and will not prompt for dependent characters until the controlling character(s) have been scored. The program will accept new taxa names from the keyboard or will read in existing names from a DELTA file. It can then be used either to create completely new descriptions or to add new characters to old descriptions which are incomplete. There is an option to print a list of unscored characters for a taxon, which can then be used as a questionnaire for observing these characters in further specimens or literature.

5.2 On-line identification programs

Those types of identification method which involve interaction with a computer while the identification of a specimen is in progress are possibly the most novel and powerful of the computerised techniques. The computer is an essential part of the method and makes possible certain techniques which cannot easily be carried out in any other way. The user, who is the biologist wanting to identify a specimen, will have a microcomputer or a computer terminal of some sort, with a keyboard for typing instructions and a visual display unit or monitor (like a television screen) for receiving the answers. There may also be a printer attached to the micro or terminal. A program is said to be *interactive*, or *on-line*, if the time between typing in an instruction or data and getting a reply is short enough to make it seem to the user that the computer is working only for him. In reality the user might be one of many working simultaneously on a microcomputer network, or with a larger *time-sharing* computer system. On the other hand one might have a microcomputer which is currently entirely occupied with, or dedicated to, the identification program. The actual computations may be taking place either centrally, locally, or both, but the degree to which the local terminal or micro is taking part in the processing may not be evident to the user.

An on-line identification program could be programmed to provide any or all of the manual identification methods described above, but designers of such programs have concentrated on those identification methods where interaction permits a step-by-step elimination or a question and answer procedure of some kind. Hence on-line programs, e.g. Boughey *et al.* (1968), Morse (1974), Pankhurst and Aitchison (1975b), Mascherpa and Bocquet (1981) and Lobanov *et al.* (1981) tend to work in a manner which is loosely related to the method of multi-access diagnostic keys, as expressed, for example, in the form of a polyclave on punched cards. In the period of time over which such programs have been developed there has been a tendency for the burden of processing to shift into the local processor (microcomputer), which now controls a whole screen of output and may include images in monochrome or colour, instead of a single output line. It has also become apparent that on-line identification programs are special cases of what are now called expert systems (see Chapter 8).

Fig. 5.1 illustrates some aspects of one such program (version 1, Pankhurst and Aitchison 1975b), using data on *Jurinea*, a genus of thistle-like plants (Kožuharov, 1976). The actual man-machine dialogue has been adapted in order to make it easier to follow. The actual program (now version 7) uses a full screen with scrolling and also colour, if the hardware permits it. Any line which was typed by the user begins with an asterisk (absent in reality) while all other output lines are displayed on a screen. Various comments have also been added, all of which are in lower case. The dialogue is initiated by the user who types various *commands*. In this program a command is a word, such as CHARACTER followed sometimes by one or more integers. Commands do not have to be typed in full, and in fact all but the first four letters are dispensed with so that, for example, CHAR is enough for CHARACTER.

Example 1 in the figure illustrates a command called BEST, which asks the machine which character is the 'best' one to use next. Ignoring considerations of cost or convenience, the computer decides this by computing the separation number (p. 191) for each character. Other criteria, such as

Fig. 5.1   An online identification session (data by Kožuharov, 1976)

Example 1

*	BEST		/Ask for the best character to begin with

SEPN	CHARACTER	
107	24 Pappus relative length	/This the best
91	16 Capitula shape	
78	10 Basal leaves hair above	/but this is easier
67	15 Capitula length	
66	17 Outer involucral bracts habit	
63	2 Stem height	
59	23 Corona of achene size	

. . . .

*	CHAR 10		/Choose character 10

10	Basal leaves hair above	
1	subglabrous above	/These are the alternative states
2	arachnoid-tomentose above	
3	setose above	

*	2		/Specimen shows state 2

9	TAXA REMAIN		
DIFFS	NO.	NAME	
0.0	1	1.J.linearifolia	/These are possible identifications
0.0	4	4.J.pinnata	
0.0	5	5.J.tanaitica	
0.0	6	6.J.albicaulis	
0.0	7	7.J.kirghisorum	
0.0	10	10.J.mollis	
0.0	14	14.J.glycacantha	
0.0	15	15.J.humilis	
0.0	16	16.J.taygetea	

*	BEST		/Ask what is the best character now

SEPN	CHARACTER
26	24 Pappus relative length
25	16 Capitula shape
21	2 Stem height
21	15 Capitula length
20	4 Stem shrubbiness

. . . .

* CHAR 15
    4 Capitula length
    0.5–7.5 cm

*	1.6–2.3		
	WELL DONE, ONE TAXON REMAINS		/Identification complete

DIFFS	NO.	NAME
0.0	4	4.J.pinnata

Example 2

*	DIAG 4		/I think it is J.pinnata

DIFFS	NO.	NAME	
130	2	Stem height	/Best diagnostic for Pinnata
130	24	Pappus relative length	
120	4	Stem shrubbiness	/but easier to use
110	16	Capitula shape	
100	23	Corona of achene size	

```
* CHAR 4
    <bleep> Character depends on 1
* CHAR   1
    1       Stem presence
    1       absent
    2       present                          /Tell the machine that there is a stem
* 2
    9       TAXA REMAIN                              /Actually the same as before
* CHAR 4                                         Describe diagnostic character
    4       stem shrubbiness
        1   herbaceous
        2   woody at base
* 2
    5       TAXA REMAIN
    DIFFS NO.   NAME
    0.0     1       1.J.linearfolia
    0.0     3       3.J.tzar-ferdinandii
    0.0     4       4.J.pinnata
    0.0     6       6.J.albicaulis
    0.0     7       7.J.kirghisorum
```

Example 3
```
* DIFF   3 4                              /How are 3 and 4 different anyhow?
    2       Stem height
            Taxon 3 = 15.0–30.0 cm
            Taxon 4 = 4.0–13.0 cm
    3       Stem leaf distribution
            Taxon 3 = 3 leafy throughout
            Taxon 4 = 1 leafless    2 leafy at base
    5       Rhizome presence
            Taxon 3 = 2 present
            Taxon 4 = 1 absent
* CHAR 3
    3       Stem leaf distribution
    1       leafless
    2       leafy at base
    3       leafy throughout
* 1/2                                  /Specimen was variable in this character
WELL DONE, ONE TAXON REMAINS
DIFFS NO.   NAME
0.0     4       4.J.pinnata
* DESC                                 /Get back a description of the specimen
    1       Stem
    1       present

    3       Stem
    1       leafless
    2       leafy at base
        . . . . . . . .
* DIFF   1                             /How does taxon 1 differ from the specimen?
    3   Stem leaf distribution                            /One difference
        Taxon 1 =   3 leafy throughout
                                    SPECIMEN = 1 leafless   2 leafy at base
    16  Capitula shape                                        /Another
```

Taxon 1 = 1 cylindrical
SPECIMEN = 4 obconical

Example 4

*	LIMI 2		/Allow up to 2 mistakes in specimen description
	14	TAXA REMAIN	
*	TAXA		

DIFFS	NO.	NAME	
2.0	1	1.J.linearifolia	/Now the number of differences
2.0	2	2.J.stoechadifolia	/between specimen and taxon shows
1.0	3	3.J.tzar-ferdinandii	
0.0	4	4.J.pinnata	
2.0	5	5.J.tanaitica	
2.0	6	6.J.albicaulis	
1.0	7	7.J.kirghisorum	
2.0	10	10.J.mollis	
2.0	12	12.J.ledebourii	
2.0	13	13.J.consanguinea	
2.0	14	14.J.glycacantha	
2.0	15	15.J.humilis	
2.0	16	16.J.taygetea	
2.0	17	17.J.fontqueri	

the information statistic, could also be used. The number (24) and name (Pappus relative length) of the currently best character are printed along with the separation (number of pairs of taxa separated by this character). Other characters with lower scores follow in a list, which may extend over several 'pages' of the screen. The machine shows that it is ready to accept a fresh command by displaying a message. It is now up to the user to pick on one of the characters suggested, whichever is the most convenient. To choose character 10 type CHAR 10, or just 10 in the most recent versions. It is also possible to type, for example,

CHAR =leaf

in order to list all characters whose names include the word 'leaf'. The machine responds by listing all the available states of this character by number and name. The program is designed this way so that the user does not need to memorise or look up which numbers correspond to which characters and states. If any of the states happen to not occur among the set of taxa currently being considered, then a question mark appears instead of the state number as a hint to the user that this state is not expected. Such states can nevertheless still be used, see below. The user now responds by typing 2 for state 2, which is what the specimen shows. Typing 1/2 would be interpreted by the machine to mean that the character was variable and both states would be remembered. If 4 had been typed, the machine would object and request another number, since state 4 does not exist. The machine now responds by listing the 9 taxa which agree with this character. The user continues by asking for another 'best' character. The answer is computed in terms of the taxa and characters currently available, i.e. the taxa which agree with the specimen as described so far and those characters which have not been used already, and which still vary. By this last is meant that characters which initially showed different states among different taxa may no longer do so once some of the taxa have been eliminated, so they become redundant for the purposes of separating the remaining taxa. How to decide which characters are the 'best' at *any* stage of the identification process is something which can only be achieved in an on-line program. Subsequently, BEST is used again and character 15, the length of the flower head, is selected. This is now a real numerical character, unlike 10, which was qualitative. There is no longer a list of states, but just a statement of the total range of variation that this character is expected to show within the current set of taxa, i.e 0.5 to 7.5 cm. The response is a range of measurements from 1.6 to 2.3, which results in the identification of the specimen as species number 4 with a congratulatory message. Note that if the user had tried to select character 10 again at this second stage, the computer would object because this character has already been used. It would also have objected if the user had tried to use a character which was currently redundant. See Example 4 for an explanation of the effect of using a state which was outside the current range of variation.

Example 2 of Fig. 5.1 shows another technique which is especially well suited to the on-line program. When asking for the 'best' character in the previous example, the user may not have had any preconceived notion as to which taxon his specimen belonged to. But suppose he had a strong suspicion that it was really a specimen of taxon 4; which characters should he use in order to prove that it is this one and not any other? This is easily answered if the taxon in question has a single diagnostic character state shown by no other taxon. Such characters are often emphasised in floras, monographs and handbooks. If, however, the specimen is incomplete and lacks the diagnostic character, or if the taxon is fairly nondescript and is distinct only by some unclear combination of several characters, an on-line program can solve this problem. The example shows the user typing DIAG 4 (for taxon number 4) and the machine gives a sequence of characters in reply, much as it did for the BEST command. Here, instead of the separation number, a diagnostic score for each character is given under the heading DIFFS. This diagnostic score is worked out as follows.

The score is of one of two different kinds, depending on the situation. If for the given taxon the character in question provides a clear-cut difference between the taxon and any of the others, the score is the number of such taxa which are different. By 'clear-cut' is meant that either the taxon has only one state for the character or, if it has several states, that none of these partially overlap with the same character on other taxa. This first kind of score is arbitrarily multiplied by a factor of 10, because it is the preferred situation. If on the other hand the character is not clear-cut, but still shows a different range of variation in the given taxon from that which it shows in others, the second score is awarded. This is just the number of taxa which show overlapping character states but which have a different range of variation possible for the taxon, so the second score is not multiplied by any factor because it refers to a potentially much less useful character.

Character 4 (shrubbiness of the stem) is selected. Other characters have higher scores, but this one is easier to use. Typing CHAR 4 results in an error message. This is because the program uses data about character dependencies to discover that not all plants have stems, and asks for this to be confirmed before proceeding. As a result of using the best diagnostic character which is suggested, number 4 with state 2, the computer finds that only 5 taxa remain; a better outcome than that obtained by using BEST, (when 9 taxa were left). The user is under no obligation to follow the suggestions of BEST or DIAG, but experience shows that an answer is reached much more quickly this way. BEST is an example of a *data-directed* strategy, where what the user chooses to do is computed from the data. On the other hand, the DIAG command is a *goal-directed* strategy, where the purpose is to prove (or disprove) that the specimen belongs to a certain taxon. It is perfectly possible to pick characters according to other criteria, or to choose them at random.

Another advantage of an on-line program is in answering some simple questions about taxa which can arise in the process of identification, but which are not always easy to answer with conventional methods. Suppose that the identification method led to one taxon as an answer, whereas one had expected it to lead to another. How then did these two differ? If the two taxa are not closely related it may not be very easy to answer this from textbooks. In example 3 of Fig. 5.1, the command DIFF 3 4 asks what are the differences between taxa numbers 3 and 4. A sequence of differing characters and their states is obtained. A similar question is answered by the next command, DIFF 1. Here the problem is to know how taxon 1 differs from the specimen so far described, because taxon 1 was thought to be a possible identification for the specimen but it has been eliminated (via other commands which are not shown). There is also an example here of variation in the specimen, where character 3 shows states 1 or 2. Variability in both specimens and taxa is commonplace, and programs must allow for it. This situation might also arise when the user is not certain which state should apply, so uncertain data can be accepted. Lastly, the command DESC is used to recall the current description of the specimen. What is shown here are really just some simple instances of *information retrieval*.

Another facility which is particularly useful in on-line programs is the *variability limit* (Morse, 1974). This is a precaution against the effect of erroneous characters in the specimen description. The computer can be told how many disagreeing characters are to be permitted. For example, if a limit of 2 is chosen, taxa will not be eliminated from the list of tentative identifications unless they have more than 2 characters in disagreement. This is shown in example 4 of Fig. 5.1. The user has entered a limit of 2 by typing LIMI 2. The machine responds by giving details on 14 taxa. Previously the machine had positively identified the specimen as taxon 4 with zero differences. In this particular program, a list of current taxa is not produced automatically unless all the taxa will fit on the screen. Another command, TAXA, is used if ever a list of taxa is needed. This list is similar to those seen earlier, but there are non-zero numbers under the column headed DIFFS (for number of characters differing). Taxon number 4 has zero differences and is first choice for the identification, but taxa 3 and 7 each have one difference and these could be checked as reasonable alternatives. One could find out where these single differences occur by typing DIFF 3 and DIFF 7. The actual number of characters in which a specimen and a taxon differ is what is shown here. Various users have suggested that character weights should be used in the on-line program, but this would have the disadvantage that the dissimilarity measure which appears as the integer number of differences would become a fractional number and this would then be less informative. A possible compromise is to present the results of commands which list characters in

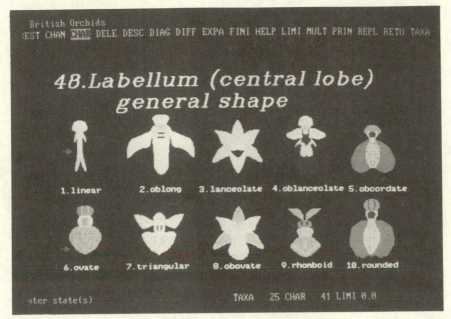

Fig. 5.2 Image of orchid character for on-line identification.

groups in the order of the character weights, which might be subjectively chosen as high, medium or low, say. This is what has been done in the Carex key (Pankhurst and Chater, 1988).

The effect of a non-zero variability limit is to create a method of identification which lies somewhere in between the sequential elimination of a diagnostic key and the method of matching by similarity coefficients. At the extreme, by setting the limit equal to the number of characters, the number of differences for each taxon will be equivalent to a dissimilarity coefficient. The higher the limit is set, the longer it will take to achieve an identification. If the limit is m, the first m characters described will not eliminate any taxa at all, and thereafter extra characters will be required if the user wants to have zero disagreements for the 'right' answer and more than m disagreements for any other, although one can choose to stop before this point. The manner in which a program such as this adjusts to errors or lack of data is sometimes called *graceful degradation*.

Finally, two simple commands which are very useful are those for replacing or deleting a character which has already been described, but which is later suspected of being wrong. Any previous character can be removed and the effect seen immediately. This is analogous to using a punched card key and taking out a card for a character which had previously been put in. In effect the key is being operated backwards when this is done.

The range of possible commands for an on-line program is very great and only some of the more characteristic ones have been described. Some interactive programs allow for weighting of characters and taxa, but this has the disadvantage that there is no longer a direct connection between the numbers of characters used and the estimate of similarity (or dissimilarity).

With modern (colour) graphic displays a considerable enhancement is possible by adding images of characters and taxa. An example is shown in Fig. 5.2, from a dataset for identification of orchids (Pankhurst, 1989). The illustration is shown in monochrome, but is actually multicoloured. Similar pictures can be provided in explanatory booklets which go with the identification program and data, but the impact of the images is very much greater when all the information is presented on the one screen, where it is very quickly retrieved. Images for this purpose can be created by means of various drawing programs, for which the so-called 'mouse' is very useful. The image in Fig. 5.2 was prepared using the Paintbrush program (Microsoft, 1985).

Since about 1980 a considerable number of new on-line identification programs have been published, e.g. Barnett, Payne and Yarrow, (1985). No attempt will be made to review all of these here, except for two particularly interesting ones. XPER by Lebbe (1984) is remarkable for its similarity to the program discussed above, in spite of being designed entirely independently. Its specifications are in the terminology of expert systems, but it is implemented in a similar fashion to that described above. Version 1 does not have an external data format such as DELTA, but has quite sophisticated editing features to allow the user to create and alter data sets. It accepts only qualitative characters. Wilson and Partridge (1986) describe ONLINEKEY, which is an on-line implementation of a diagnostic key. The program decides which couplet is to be used next. Morse (1974) mentions the same idea, but dismisses it in favour of leaving the user with full freedom to choose characters. Other on-line programs have intentionally not included a *control system* such as this. ONLINEKEY is also interesting because it includes a learning procedure (Section 1.5). More work is needed in this area because experience in a project for a polyclave to grasses (Pankhurst and Allinson, 1985) has shown that uncritical acceptance of data from named specimens leads to the inclusion of much aberrant character data and the blurring of vital distinctions between taxa. An algorithm is needed to determine what is valid variation and what is not.

A recent version of the on-line key is INTKEY, which is bundled with the DELTA data set on world grass genera (Watson and Dallwitz, 1988). This has been developed with large data sets in mind, and in this particular application, handles 765 taxa and 469 characters. INTKEY was developed out of version 3 of the Pankhurst and Aitchison on-line program, with additional features. It does not have full-screen working or graphics but has other extra features:

1) It can be used in either an identification mode or an information retrieval mode (see p. 13). The difference is in fact not very great, and hinges on the treatment of missing and overlapping data. If a character of a taxon is unknown, that taxon should not be eliminated when that character is used in identification. On the other hand, a taxon should be eliminated during retrieval if the desired character is not positively recorded. There are features to combine characters with 'and' and 'or' in searches for taxa. In particular, it is possible to search for taxa which do not have a given character state.

2) There are options to include and exclude particular taxa and characters, which is useful for a large data set. The DELTA format already has directives for this purpose. There is an option to cut down the number of characters examined by the BEST command, since this may take a long time with a large data set.

3) Character weightings (reliabilities) can optionally be used in calculating similarities and dissimilarities.

4) There is a command to list the similarities between taxa as well as the differences, and a command for finding diagnostic descriptions (see p. 154).

5.3 Key-constructing programs

A number of computer programs exist which can construct diagnostic keys, e.g. Dallwitz (1974), Hall (1973), Morse (1974), Pankhurst (1970 and 1971), Payne (1975), Ross (1975) and Lobanov *et al.* (1981). In what follows only *batch* mode programs are discussed, i.e. programs which once started, run without consulting the user again. Interactive key construction is discussed in a later section (p. 132). In the terminology of computer science, an identification key would be called a *decision tree*, and there have been efforts by workers outside taxonomy to produce something very similar, e.g. Quinlan (1979 and 1985). The following account does not describe the workings of any of these in particular, but gives a general account of the methods and options. This is because development in this field is very rapid and improvements are being made all the time, so that any statement of what a particular program could or could not do would be unreliable.

5.3.1 Program logic

The general sequence of events in constructing a key in a computer is now described. To begin with the data matrix and its associated information is read into store. What happens after this point is broadly similar to the procedure for constructing keys manually (p. 92). At the start all taxa and characters are potentially available, apart from some taxa or characters which may be weighted in some special way in order to show that they are not to be used at all. Note is kept throughout of which taxa are being considered and which characters are applicable to them. Even at the beginning some characters may be redundant. This can be detected by the fact that they show the same state or states throughout or have all the states missing. Special considerations apply to dependent characters. Since such a character cannot be used before its controlling character (e.g. 'wing presence' must come before 'wing length'), keys are not allowed to begin with dependent characters.

Suppose for the moment that all characters and taxa have equal weight; the next task is to choose a character from among those available. This is done by calculating some figure of merit which measures the suitability of each character for forming a question in the key. The details of this are given below (p. 127), but when this figure has been calculated for every character, the character which has the best score is the one chosen. It is then possible to decide how many leads this key branch will have by counting the number of different states or combinations of states which occur, and to make a list of which taxa show each of these. The program could also consider more than one character at a time, as two or more could be taken together. The chances of finding neat ways of branching a key with several characters in a question decrease rapidly with the number of characters involved, while the computing time (and cost) increases rapidly. Hence it is wise to control the search for multiple character leads in some way, and this can be done by putting an upper limit to the number of characters allowed. The construction of the key branch is not quite complete, because there may be useful auxiliary characters. To find these, use the lists of taxa which go in each lead of the branch, and consider whether there are any characters which vary in exact correlation with the principal character(s). Such characters will have a state which is the same within the taxa in each lead but which is different between at least some of the different leads. If any auxiliary characters are found, they must be remembered along with the primary character(s). This is now the moment to sort the leads into an order of increasing size and to store away the details of the key branch which has just been created in computer memory. This same method of finding auxiliary characters is also described by Payne (1980).

Auxiliary characters, if they can be found, are also a means of guarding against errors when the key is used. If a user of a key misreads a character of a specimen, the result may still be correct if the key obliges him to consider other characters before reaching a conclusion. Payne and Preece (1977) describe an option to a key construction program which insists on a given minimum number of character differences (a variability limit) for a taxon before it is keyed out. They also suggest that a *check key* could be constructed for each taxon, so that after the taxon is keyed out in the normal way, a secondary key be used to re-examine the specimen. The check key for a taxon includes all the taxa which differ from it by up to as many characters as the limit is set to, and uses characters which have not been used in the main key as far as possible.

Subsequent questions and leads are generated in much the same way in a suitable sequence, but with a reduced set of taxa and characters as appropriate. A suitable sequence of leads could be that of a parallel key or of a yoked key (p. 88). This can also be regarded as a process of crossing out some rows and columns of the data matrix. The character(s) which are used as primary characters in a branch cannot be used again in derived branches further down. On the other hand, it may be useful to get the program to use the same characters repeatedly in different parts of the key as far as possible, so that the total number of different characters required is reduced (see Payne, 1975). If there is a definite cost associated with characters, e.g. as with tests on bacteria, this can be an advantage. The use of character weights will also tend to reduce the total number of characters used by favouring those which have high weights. The characters which are now available may not all be useful since, among the reduced set of taxa, some of them may be temporarily redundant. This procedure is repeated until every lead terminates with a single taxon, or there are no more characters which separate taxa.

If characters have different weights, there are several ways to take account of this. One is to group the characters according to weight and only consider those characters which are available which belong to the group of the highest occurring weight. This will ensure that characters are used in descending order of weight, providing that the distribution of states among taxa permits them to be used at all. Another way to use character weights is to include them in the figure of merit discussed below. A special case is a weight, for example a negative weight, which indicates that a character is not to be used at all.

5.3.2 The figure of merit

The figure of merit, also called a separation function, is devised in order to decide between different possible ways of branching a key. The figure is heuristic, which means that it is justified only by the fact that it works, and not necessarily by theory. It represents a compromise between the various qualities that a 'good' key question should have and is a combination of various factors. The figure of merit can be arranged to have the highest value for the 'best' question, so that the scores for the various characters or combinations of characters are searched for the largest score. It can just as well be arranged to give the smallest score for the 'best' branch, and that is how it will be presented here.

(a) *The information given by a character*. For this purpose, the separation coefficient, s, or the information statistic, I, can be used (see p. 191). These both increase for better characters, and can be made to suit by subtracting from the maximum value. Since both can be arranged to vary between 0 and 1, one could use $(1-s)$ or $(1-I)$ which will then be smallest for the best character. Both can be adapted to cover several characters in combination and can be used on any kind of character. The separation coefficient is perhaps simpler to calculate and has a more obvious interpretation.

The above is easiest to apply when all taxa show only one state for a character. If some taxa show variable states for a character, the separation coefficient is still straightforward to apply, because even when there is variation, the question, 'Does this character distinguish this pair of taxa?' can still be answered. The information statistic can be used in this case if the proportion of each state occurring for a variable character within each taxon is known (Payne, 1975).

(b) *Dichotomies*. If the number of different character states or combinations of states is K, the question will have K leads. K equals two (dichotomous branching) is usually preferred. Any function of K which increases rapidly for K greater than two would do. One could take a power, e.g. $(K-2)^2$ or $(K-2)^3$, or take an exponential function, e.g. $\exp(K-2)$. Such functions would discourage anything other than dichotomous branches.

(c) *Equal numbers of taxa in leads*. The best arrangement is to have the same number of taxa in every lead. If there are K leads, let the numbers of taxa be n_1, n_2, up to n_K, so that the total is N.

$$\sum_{i=1}^{K} n_i = N$$

If all these were equal, then for any i, $n_i = N/K$. Usually the n_i are not all the same so that

$$\left(n_i - \frac{N}{K} \right)$$

is the difference between the ideal and the actual. In order to remove the effect of a different number of taxa at different stages of the key, it would be better to consider

$$\left(1 - \frac{N}{n_i K} \right)$$

This is either positive or negative, so it could be squared to make it always positive or else the minus sign could just be removed (signified by vertical lines), viz:

$$\left(1 - \frac{N}{n_i K}\right)^2 \quad \text{or} \quad \left|1 - \frac{N}{n_i K}\right|$$

This could be added together for all leads, e.g.

$$\sum_{i=1}^{K} \left(1 - \frac{N}{n_i K}\right)^2$$

This figure would tend to be larger for larger values of K, and if this effect is not wanted, one could divide by K. In this way we have found a function which will be zero for the ideal and increases for any other arrangement.

If taxa have been given different weights, it is here that this can take effect. This can most easily be done by treating a weighted taxon of weight w as if it were represented w times. If w is 10 for one taxon, for example, then a key branch with this taxon on its own in one lead would exactly balance 10 other taxa each with weight 1 in another lead. Hence the heavily weighted taxon can be keyed out separately at an earlier stage. The above formula is altered by replacing n_i by n'_i where n'_i is the sum of the weights of the taxa in lead i instead of just the number of taxa. Likewise N becomes N' where the weights of all taxa are added and not just their total number taken.

(d) *Missing character states.* It is preferable not to use characters whose states are missing from the definitions of the taxa. This is because any taxon whose state is unknown for a character that is to be used in a key branch, has to be put in all the leads in case someone observes the character later. This increases the size of the key and contributes nothing to the identification of the taxon. Sometimes, e.g. with fossils, characters of taxa are often missing and such characters are hard to avoid. In this case, it may be better not to try and make a key but to use a different identification method instead (see p. 160).

Suppose we have a binary character with some missing states. If the number of taxa with state 1 is n_1, with state 2 is n_2 and with n_0 missing, then

$$n_0 + n_1 + n_2 + = N$$

The numbers of taxa, effectively, with states 1 and 2 will be

$$n'_1 = n_1 + n_0$$
$$\text{and } n'_2 = n_2 + n_0$$

since the missing states could occur equally well as 1 or 2, or both, as far as is known. The new values of n'_1 and n'_2 can be used in the formula under (c) for testing equal distributions of taxa as before. To discourage the expansion of missing states, the proportion

$$r = \frac{n_0}{N}$$

could be used in the figure of merit or, for a more severe deterrent, just the value n_0.

(e) *Quantitative characters.* There is a special situation which occurs with quantitative characters. One could have two quantitative characters which were equally good in all respects as above but which still differ in the degree to which they separate the taxa. For example, suppose there are two characters A (range 0-50) and B (range 20-200). Which would be better for separating taxa X and Y, if the states are as follows?

	A	B
X	0–15	150–200
Y	35–50	20–90

The gap in the values of A is 20 (between 15 and 35) and for B is 60 (150 minus 90). Is B therefore better, because the gap is larger, and thereby making a clearer distinction? Not necessarily, because B varies more. It would be better to find the ratio of the gap to the total range, which for A is 20/50 = 0.4 and for B is 60/180 = 0.33. Hence, on this count, A is really the better choice. This ratio increases for better characters, so to put it in the same manner as the other figures we could use

$$1 - \frac{\text{gap}}{\text{total range}}$$

A character of this kind is said to be *bimodal*, and a measure such as the above is used by Hall (1973). A bimodal character could arise with variable qualitative characters which have many states, but this would be a rare situation.

(f) *Character weight.* This could be treated as contributing to the figure of merit as a separate item. If so, it would need to be put in a form such as

$$(\text{maximum weight - weight})$$

$$\text{or} \quad \frac{1}{\text{weight}} \quad \text{or} \quad \exp(-\text{weight})$$

so that the best character makes the smallest contribution.

Finally these figures can be combined into one figure of merit in various ways. They could just be added together, or they could be multiplied by a positive constant before being added together, in order to alter the relative importance given to different aspects of 'goodness' of characters. The figures could also be multiplied together or some could be added and others multiplied into the final figure. One arrangement which would be particularly sensible would be to add together figures (a) to (e) and then multiply by a factor for the character weight. A comparison of some different figures of merit for key construction is given by Gower and Payne (1975), with special reference to the effect of missing characters. Brown (1977) shows that there is a wide class of functions which are suitable. Payne (1981) investigated which criteria lead to the most efficient keys in different circumstances, and Payne and Dixon (1984) measured their efficiency in simulation experiments. They found that no one criterion performed consistently better than any other, and that the differences in the expected cost of identification were not normally very great.

5.3.3 Programming details

A number of rather more special details are covered here, including some points of interest to computer programmers.

(a) *Partial keys.* The usual way to recognise that a key branch has been completed is when all taxa are distinct and the final leads each relate to one taxon only. If in fact all the taxa were not distinct from each other, this could be regarded as an error in the data matrix. Occasionally an incomplete or partial key may actually be desired, in which case the branching of the key may terminate with more than one taxon in a lead. The reason for stopping may be that there are no characters left by which taxa could be separated.

(b) *Duplicate taxon names.* Usually all the names of taxa in the database will be different, but occasionally several forms of one taxon will all be described under one name. In this case the branching of the key must cease as soon as all the taxa in a lead have the same name, even if there are several and even if there are still characters available. As an example of this, a data matrix might include species from several genera. If the species all had different names, a key to the species could be made, but if only their generic names were given, a generic key would result.

(c) *Unusual taxa.* Programs for key construction could be written which attempt to identify taxa which are 'unusual'. This would require estimating what the description of an average taxon would be, and finding those which are least similar beyond some arbitrary limit. Even so this would not guarantee that the 'unusual' taxa would always have some convenient diagnostic characters for separating them. The easiest course seems to be simply to decide subjectively which the 'unusual' taxa are and to give high weightings to their diagnostic characters, which will have the desired effect. If there are no obvious diagnostic characters, taxon weighting could be used to give these taxa prominence, provided that suitable distributions of character states exist. There does not seem to be any particular need to write program statements specifically to deal with 'unusual' taxa.

(d) *Variation of characters within taxa.* A method of describing characters in the data matrix which permits any variation to be included within a coding of one integer number has already been described (p. 113). This may have appeared awkward but is conveniently arranged for the internal logic of computers. Integer numbers are stored as a sum of powers of two, and hence a state recorded, as in the previous example, where the number 25 is stored as

$$16 + 8 + 1,$$

or

$$1.16 + 1.8 + 0.4 + 0.2 + 1.1$$

which is

$$1.2^4 + 1.2^3 + 0.2^2 + 0.2^1 + 1.2^0$$

This is stored as the binary number 11001, where the 0's and 1's are just the multipliers from in front of the powers of two. Practically every digital computer is provided with two simple instructions, called a logical sum and a logical difference. The logical sum of two numbers is a pattern of 0's and 1's, such that there is a 1 if both the corresponding positions are 1, and 0 otherwise. This is in fact the answer to the question, 'Have these two taxa any states in common for this character, and if so, which?' Likewise the logical difference answers the question, 'What are the states shown by one or other or both of two taxa for this character?' The use of this internal representation for characters is therefore very convenient for answering questions such as these within a program, regardless of whether the characters vary or not.

(e) *Internal storage of keys.* While a computer is constructing a key, it has to store the partly completed version in its memory in order to be able to find out which taxa and characters are appropriate to each new branch. A convenient way to do this is to use what is called a *list structure*. That is to say, while the details about the leads of any one question are kept together in consecutive words of the store, called a *block*, the different blocks are scattered throughout part of the store which is called a *free storage* area. A record is kept of how large each block is, and where it is. Special subroutines permit the program to 'ask' for blocks of suitable size when they are needed, and to relinquish them later when they are no longer required. The need to 'give up' blocks of store can arise when a question is constructed but is replaced by a better question found subsequently. The list structure also contains *pointers*, which means that a note is kept within each block saying where the next one is. These pointers are like the lines joining the boxes in the tree diagram of a key in Fig. 1.3. In this context, the 'next' block is the one which corresponds to the next question which would be written on the page when the key is expressed in words. There are therefore two ways of ordering the blocks, according to whether the sequence of a parallel or yoked key is used. This can be described another way by saying that the order for a parallel key corresponds to tracing out the tree of the key (Fig. 1.3) across the levels from left to right before moving down the levels and that the order for a yoked key is from top to bottom before left to right. A useful way of keeping track of a partly completed key is to use what is called a *stack*. This means keeping a note of which was the last block considered at each level, and a note of the current level number.

While in most key-constructing programs it is convenient to use a list structure for storing the key, it is not essential to do so. Dallwitz (1974) stores the key as a rectangular table which is written on top of the initial data matrix of taxa and characters.

(f) *Printing of keys.* Some programs print the key in a numerical form which can then be written out by hand to give a finished product. Others go on to print the text of the key. This basically means substituting words for the numerical version of the key, plus laying it out neatly on paper. A parallel key, or else a yoked key, is obtained merely by choosing one of the two alternative ways of following the list structure (see last section). If indentation is required, this is easily found from the level of each key branch in the tree (Fig. 1.3). If the question is at level L, it must be moved (L-1) spaces to the right. The program will distinguish between leads which end in the names of taxa and those which point to other leads. Punctuation with commas and full stops must be inserted and, if a sentence is too long for the width of a page, it must be broken between two words and continued on the next line. It used to be the case that computers could only print upper case (capital) letters, but nowadays lower case (small) letters are usually available, and can be put in as appropriate. Further sophistication can be obtained by attending to the left to right order of characters in multicharacter leads, e.g. for flowering plants it is customary to follow a sequence of vegetative, then floral and finally fruiting characters when writing a description. However, the principal character must still come first. Information to describe this desired order would then need to be added to the data format, which was not included in the above discussion. It is also possible to improve the phrasing of the sentences by removing repeated words, e.g. the phrase

Wings present, wings 5-10 mm long

could be simplified to

Wings present, 5-10 mm long.

More recent developments in the field of computing and publications allow the possibility of computerised typesetting and desktop publishing. It is now possible to include different fonts of different sizes, to have proportional spacing of the letters, to specify the layout of the document on the page and to include pictures and diagrams, all under computer control. To put this another way, the output from the key program can now include data or instructions in addition to the actual text, which specify how the document is to be printed. Several of the authors of key-constructing programs have experimented with computer typesetting, e.g. Dallwitz (1984) and Payne (1984). Desktop publishing programs are now available for microcomputers which produce a similar result, but they use laser printers to give immediate camera-ready copy which can then be used directly for printing by photographic methods. Unfortunately, there is not as yet any standard way of expressing the printing instructions.

5.4 Interactive key construction

An interactive key-construction program is possibly the ideal means of writing diagnostic keys. The program can take care of all the storage and retrieval of the necessary facts and carry out all the bookkeeping aspects of writing a key, but leaves the user, i.e. the taxonomic expert, to make good choices of characters based on his experience. More than this, the program can also help the user to discover what the best choices are. The design of such a program follows naturally from the previous discussion of on-line identification programs and batch mode key-construction programs. The discussion centres on the program KCONI (Pankhurst, 1988b).

Batch mode key-constructing programs have been in use for as long as twenty years, but have not found universal acceptance. Evidence has accumulated that keys produced by batch methods are still regarded as being less than ideal. This is not merely to say that after the program has run, the output key has to be further edited and polished with a word processor, in order to add minor detail, and to improve the style. This would be true for any computer-constructed key. Rather, what is meant is that the key is not exactly the kind of key which an expert would have chosen to write, had it been written by hand. Taxonomic experts prefer to make subjective choices of characters at every stage, and do not particularly want to have a consistent algorithm for these decisions. The discussion attached to the review of Payne and Preece (1980) shows that taxonomists, mathematicians and computer programmers differ on this point. The purpose of an interactive key-constructing program is therefore not to increase mathematical refinement in the algorithms but to increase participation by the taxonomic expert.

The use of batch mode key-construction programs offers many advantages. It is very easy to alter the controls on the data, such as the weights attached to taxa and characters, in order to produce a new key with a different emphasis. It is also quite simple to produce the key in different output styles, to alter the data by adding, removing or changing taxa and characters, and to generate a new key afterwards. In spite of this, there are desirable features of keys which such programs do not provide, or cannot provide easily.

The main advantage of interactive key construction is (1) The freedom with which the taxonomic expert can choose exactly whichever character(s) are preferred at every stage. Further advantages include the following: (2) There is at every stage a choice of strategy between keying all taxa or trying to key particular taxa, or just making a subjective character choice; (3) When there are more than two states available in a character, these can be recombined in different ways. Likewise, if a potential lead contains more than two questions, these can be recombined to enforce a dichotomy; (4) When there are taxa which have only relative differences (see p. 95) in the available characters, and only a partial key is possible, the expert can decide whether and how far to continue. These points are discussed in detail below.

1) Choice of characters. Whilst an expert may be expected to select the 'best' character(s) at every stage, this can be interpreted in several ways, such that a compromise is necessary. The character might be the most efficient in terms of information content for constructing an optimum key, or it could be the most diagnostic for a particular taxon, or it might be a character which is significant in the classification. It might be the one which is easiest to observe accurately, or the one most likely to be visible in a preserved specimen, or what is most likely to be available in the field. It may not be possible to combine all these factors into a simple and convenient formula, as required in the automatic key programs.

2) Different strategies. In the batch programs for key construction it has been usual to seek an optimal key at every stage. In the terminology of expert systems, this is a 'data-directed' strategy, i.e. it is assumed that we do not know which particular taxon is being sought in the key, and so we try to allow equally well for all possibilities. However, it has long been customary when writing keys manually to deliberately arrange the key so that 'unusual' taxa come out near the beginning. This strategy is the opposite of the last, since the idea is to diagnose a particular taxon, and separate it from all the rest. This is a 'goal-directed' strategy, and is unlikely to be optimal for the key as a whole. Nevertheless, a taxonomist might well prefer to be permitted to use either strategy (or neither!) wherever it seems most appropriate. Another point is that it is well known, e.g. Payne (1975) that a heuristic function may make choices which are optimal only for one lead of the key, but not at all optimal when a larger section of the key is considered as a whole. It is not very practical in a batch program to explore many levels of leads at once because of the time required. In an interactive program, however, it is possible to explore the alternatives locally within the key when this difficulty arises.

3) Recombination of states and questions. If the data contains only binary characters, then this question does not arise. However, it is probably no longer reasonable to expect taxonomists to restrict their characters to binary form only, and multistate characters are part and parcel of the DELTA format, which is now in general use. If multistate characters occur in the data, then leads with more than two questions may occur in the key. This might or might not be considered acceptable. Consider the *Epilobium* character 'Plant <habit>' with states 'prostrate', 'decumbent to ascending' and 'more or less erect'. A lead based on this might use three questions:

Plant prostrate
Plant decumbent to ascending
Plant more or less erect

but this might be better with just two questions, as

> Plant prostrate or decumbent to ascending
> Plant more or less erect

or as

> Plant prostrate
> Plant decumbent to ascending or more or less erect

Which of these is going to be the most suitable? The example can be made more complex by having several characters together in the lead. There is no easy means to resolve this except in the interactive program, where states of characters can be grouped and questions recombined.

4)   Partial keys. Consider two species with two characters which are only relatively different as follows:

Species A. Stigma shorter than or about equal to style,
            flowers 6 to 10mm diameter,
Species B. Stigma shorter than style,
            flowers 6 to 15mm diameter,

where a key using flower characters is wanted, and there are no other convenient characters in which these species differ absolutely. The lead could just terminate here with the two species names at the end of a question. However, some specimens could still be distinguished if we write:

1 Stigma about equal style	Species A
Stigma shorter than style	2
2 Flowers over 10mm diameter	Species B
Flowers 6 to 10 mm diameter	Species A or B

An interactive key program can allow the taxonomist to decide what best to do in this type of situation, whether and how far to continue and when to terminate.

There is one possible disadvantage of the interactive method, which is that it is not as easy to make alterations to the data and then to build the key again. The KCONI program has been written so that, for a given data file, an existing key can be repeatedly revised by deleting any lead or leads, and can be printed out in various forms. If the taxonomic data file is changed, however, it may be necessary to build the key from the beginning again, depending on the number and complexity of the changes. Evidently, if only a few characters are changed which are only used in terminal leads of the key, the revision can be made by word processing alone, but if the first lead is to use different characters, then the key will be entirely new. It is not obvious how an interactive program could be written which could revise a given key with changed taxon and character definitions. A much simpler alternative is to arrange for a batch key program to process the new data file in the normal way to produce a key and to transfer this new key in numerical form into the interactive program for further revisions, which is what has been done.

In order to give an idea of how an interactive key-constructing program operates, some notes on the use of KCONI follow below. It is possible either to start on a new key, or to read back one which already exists and which may or may not be already complete.

1)   KCONI chooses an unfinished branch of the key to work on.

2) The expert makes a selection of character(s) which could be used to build the next lead, or asks the program for advice on which character(s) to use.

3) The user explores various alternatives for the next lead and eventually decides to adopt one of them, which KCONI stores.

4) Repeat from 1) until the key is complete, or view any part of the key as built so far, or delete any part or parts of it, and then repeat. The partly finished or complete key can be saved on file at any time. Finally, print the key.

This will now be considered in more detail. The program begins by considering all available taxa and characters. Each character is checked to see that:

1) it has not been excluded by deliberate weighting in the data;

2) it has not been used already, or if it has been used in an earlier lead on which the new lead depends, then it was variable there, e.g. if earlier on, leaflet shape was included in a question which stated 'leaflets elliptic or ovate', it might now be possible to use 'leaflets elliptic' and 'leaflets ovate' in different questions;

3) it is not redundant, in the sense that there are at least two current taxa for which the character shows contrasting states;

4) it is not dependent on another character, or if it is, that the controlling character has already been used in an earlier lead with state(s) which permit it to occur here, e.g. if the character is 'Stem hairs spreading' then 'Stem hairs present' must have been used previously, because if only taxa for which 'Stem hairs absent' are being considered, then the character is illegal.

There are then three different ways in which character(s) for the lead may be selected. The commands referred to below have already been described for the on-line identification program (p. 117). Examples of the program in use are shown in Fig. 5.3. The command CHAR could be used to see which characters are available, and a subjective choice made. On the other hand, if a more or less optimal key is wanted, the command BEST is used to find which characters are the most divisive, or else the command DIAG could be used to find characters which will diagnose a particular taxon. The program presents different ordered lists of characters according to the strategy chosen. Another command which can help with making questions out of multi-state characters is EXPAnd, which shows the distribution of states of a character among the current taxa. Lastly, if there are relatively few taxa in the lead, the DIFF command can be used to display exactly which characters distinguish two taxa.

The most important and most complex command is called EXAM, and allows one or more characters to be tried out with a view to constructing the next lead. The number of questions generated depends on the number of states available in the characters chosen, so that if for example, a two-state and a three-state character are selected, there could be as many as six questions. In practice there may be fewer, since not all the combinations of states may actually occur, and because more than one combination of states may apply to the same group of taxa, in which case the characters are merged before the question is displayed. Any taxa for which a character is missing are simply assigned to every question. Each question is numbered and shown in turn, with all the characters and states spelt out and numbered. If any auxiliary characters exist which correlate with the principal character(s), these are

Fig. 5.3   Example of interactive key construction using *Epilobium*
(i)   Begin key, 13 taxa, 17 characters available, command BEST.
     Sepn   Characters
     52   13 Flower diameter
     42   10 Stem leaves shape at base
     42   16 Stigma length relative to style
     40   17 Calyx tube glandular hairs
     . . . .
(ii) Try first lead with EXAM 16
1   (16) Stigma (=1) shorter than style.
     TAXA 2 3 4 6 10 11 12
2   (16) Stigma (=2) about equal style.
     TAXA 1 5 7 8 9 13
This will be lead number 1
Accept (A), abandon (Q) display again (D)? A

(iii) 6 taxa and 16 characters; BEST again, then EXAM 13
     Sepn   Characters
     12   13 Flower diameter
     11   14 Flower colour
      9   17 Calyx tube glandular hairs
      8   4 Stem glandular hairs
      8   9 Stem leaves decurrent
      8   10 Stem leaves shape at base
      8   11 Leaves shiny
     . . . .
1 (13) Flower diameter 3.0 to 5.5 mm, (+9) stem leaves (=1) not
decurrent.   TAXA 5 13
2 (13) Flower diameter 6.0 to 9.0 mm, (+9) stem leaves
(=2) decurrent.   TAXA 7 9
3 (13) Flower diameter 10.0 to 23.0 mm, (+9) stem leaves
(=) decurrent.   TAXA 1 8
Type D, N, O, Q, R, S or T

(iv)   Recombine questions 2 and 3, new character order 9 and 13 and use T
command to see taxon names
1 (+9) Stem leaves (=1) not decurrent, (13) flower diameter 3.0 to 5.5mm.
          TAXA 5 13
             5 E.roseum
            13 E.brunnescens
2 (+9) Stem leaves (=2) decurrent, (13) flower diameter 6.0 to 23.0 mm.
          TAXA 1 7 8 9
This will be lead number 2

(v)   2 taxa and 8 characters, BEST (not shown) and EXAM 1
1   (1) Plant (=1) prostrate, (+4) stem (=1) without glandular hairs, (+6) stem (=2)
rooting at nodes, (+10) stem leaves (=2) rounded at base, (+12) flowers (=1)
axillary, (+14) flower (=2) pink, (+17) calyx tube (=1) without glandular hairs, (+18)
fruit stalk 2.5 to 6.0 cm.
     13. E.brunnescens
2   (1) Plant (=3) more or less erect, (+4) stem (=2) with glandular hairs, (+6) stem
(=1) not rooting at nodes, (+10) stem leaves (=1) cuneate at base, (+12) flowers
(=2) terminal, (+14) flower (=1) white to pale pink, (+17) calyx tube (=2) with
glandular hairs, (+18) fruit stalk 0.5 to 1.9 cm.
     5. E.roseum
Type D, N, O, Q, R, S or T

(vi)   Delete characters 4, 14, 17 and 18
1 (1) Plant (=1) prostrate, (+6) stem (=2) rooting at nodes, (+10) stem leaves (=2) rounded at base, (+12) flowers (=1) axillary.
    13. E.brunnescens
2 (1) Plant (=3) more or less erect, (+6) stem (=1) not rooting at nodes, (+10) stem leaves (=1) cuneate at base, (+12) flowers (=2) terminal.
    5. E.roseum
This will be lead number 3

(vii)   VIEW the key so far.
1 Stigma about equal style.   2
  Stigma shorter than style.   0
2 Stem leaves not decurrent, flower diameter 3.0 to 5.5 mm   3
  Stem leaves decurrent, flower diameter 6.0 to 23.0 mm   0
3 Plant prostrate, stem rooting at nodes, stem leaves rounted at base,
  flowers axillary.   13. E.brunnescens
  Plant more or less erect, stem not rooting at nodes, stem leaves cuneate
  at base, flowers terminal.   5. E.roseum

(viii)   New key, DIAG 13, then EXAM 1 6 12

DIFFS	NO.	NAME
120	12	Flowers position
120	6	Stem rooting at nodes
120	1	Plant habit
100	18	Fruit stalk length

      . . . . . .
1 (1) Plant (=1) prostrate, (6) stem (=2) rooting at nodes, (12) flowers (= 1) axillary.
           13. E.brunnescens
2 (1) Plant (=2) decumbent to ascending or (=3) more or less erect, (6) stem (=1) not rooting at nodes, (12) flowers (=2) terminal.
      TAXA 1 2 3 4 5 6 7 8 9 10 11 12
This will be lead number 1
Accept (A), abandon (Q) display again (D)? A

inserted automatically, but are marked with a + (plus sign). Under each question there is a list of the taxa which belong there, or else the name of the taxon if there is only one. There are a number of subsidiary options which permit the lead to be explored and edited. The usual procedure is to look through the questions one by one (option Next). After the last question the lead can be accepted, abandoned, or redisplayed. After each question there are the following options:

    Next, to see the next question,
    Quit, to abandon the EXAM command altogether,
    Skip, to jump to the last question, without quitting,
    Taxa, to list the names of the taxa in the current question,
    Delete, to remove any unwanted auxiliary characters,
    Recombine, to combine any of the questions together, and,
    Order, to change the order of the characters within questions.

    Auxiliary (confirmatory) characters are always searched for and inserted, so that if none appear, this means that none exist. Such characters are found by examining the unused current characters within the taxon groups in the questions to find out whether the combined states within those groups are distinct in every group. Notice, however, that the program does not detect auxiliary characters which are not exact. It is not programmed to produce phrases with qualifications such as 'often' or 'usually'. If any or all of the auxiliary characters are unwanted, then they can be deleted with the Delete option.

The Recombine option is important because it allows the whole lead to be recast. There are various reasons for doing this. One reason is that the expert may want to make this lead into a dichotomy. Another is that merging the states of multi-state characters might make a better lead (see the example given above). Also, if the chosen character(s) are variable or missing in some of the taxa, then some of the taxa may have been repeated too often in the different questions, which will be visible from the displayed lists of taxon numbers. After the user has typed R the program asks for two question numbers and then joins those two questions together, merging the character states and the lists of taxa. The auxiliary characters also have to be reassigned, since they may now be different. The order of the characters within the lead can also be changed, as it may be desired to have vegetative characters before those of flower and fruit, for example. This process of recombining questions and deleting and reordering characters can be repeated as often as desired.

A worked example based on *Epilobium* is shown in Fig. 5.3. The figure does not show the full-screen layout actually used. (i)To begin with, it is assumed that an optimal key is wanted, so that the BEST command is used. For simplicity, BEST is used to seek a new lead based on a single character, although it can in fact be used to explore two or more characters simultaneously. (ii)A lead using character 16 is explored. It produces two alternatives carrying almost equal numbers of taxa and without duplication of any taxa between the two questions. For convenience, the character and state numbers are shown in this display although they are dropped when the key is printed later. This lead is accepted as lead number 1 of the key. (iii)The program automatically selects one of the incomplete branches of lead 1 and shows that here there are now 6 taxa with 16 characters to distinguish them. BEST is used again and character 13 is EXAMined. Character 13 is quantitative (flower diameter) but has been divided into suitable ranges with the KEY STATES directive in DELTA (p.115) so that three questions are proposed. In addition, the auxiliary character 9 (stem leaves decurrent) has been found. Supposing that a dichotomous key is required, this lead is not satisfactory as it stands. (iv)The options for revising the lead are used to recombine questions 2 and 3, and also to reverse the order of the characters 13 and 9 in order to put the stem character before the flower character. At the same time the program has merged the flower diameter range from questions 2 and 3. After the first question the T option was used in order to see the names of the taxa. (v)After accepting the previous lead, just two taxa are left in one of the key branches. EXAMination of character 1 gives a dichotomous lead with 7 auxiliary characters in which two individual species are keyed out. Not all these characters are equally useful, and the questions are perhaps unnecessarily long, so in (vi) four of these characters are deleted in order to make the questions shorter. In (vii) the VIEW command is used to display the key as constructed so far. References to leads which have not yet been completed are shown as zeros. The style of key used here is not necessarily the one chosen for the final print of the complete key. The process of key construction is abandoned at this point in order to show the effect of a different strategy. In (viii) we begin again with the intention of keying out species 13 before the others. This species is an introduction and is strikingly different in appearance from the native species. The DIAG command is used to find diagnostic characters for it. Three characters are shown to have the same diagnostic value, so all three are used together in the EXAM command. The lead which results has a neat dichotomy which distinguishes species 13 from all the others and contains three correlated characters. It will not always happen that character state distributions exist which will give such a neat resolution as this.

A complication which may occur is when it happens that only a partial key is possible at the current lead, as in the example given previously. The program then gives the option either to continue, and to build more leads with characters which only partially differentiate the taxa, or else to simply terminate the lead with the names of the remaining taxa. This option is offered repeatedly if there are several such partial characters, until either all characters are used, or else a decision is made to terminate this part of the key. At any stage, the key as built so far, or any part of it, can be shown on the display with the VIEW command. This version of the key is always shown in the yoked form, and unfinished leads are numbered with zeros. Similarly, it is possible at any time to use the SAVE command in order to save the key on a file, in a numerical form, so that it can be called back later for further processing, or so that it can be printed.

When the key is complete, and there are no more leads which need to be built, a message is displayed. At this point, it is possible to delete any of the leads in the key with the DELE command. It does not matter whether the key has been freshly created, or whether it has been saved and then read back in again, but it does have to be complete. If the lead which is to be deleted has other leads depending on it, then all the dependent leads are deleted as well. If the lead(s) happen to be at the end of the key, then the last lead number is amended. Otherwise, the total number of leads remains the same, but one or several lead numbers or sequences of lead numbers disappear. The normal process of creating new leads then begins again, until the key is once more complete. Since a printed version of the older version of the key is likely to be on hand, and being used as a basis for the revision, the original undeleted lead numbers are maintained during this process, and when new leads are created, they are assigned numbers which begin after the previous highest number. When this revised key is complete, it is now necessary to renumber all the leads, and the RENU command is used for this. Finally, the saved key can be printed, with a choice of two styles, parallel or yoked, with or without indentation, and with a choice of page width.

5.5 Punched card keys

Punched card keys, their construction and their uses, have already been described (see p. 101). The universal punched card which used to be used by computers had 80 columns and 12 rows and was body-punched across its

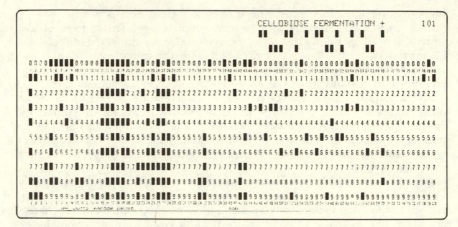

Fig. 5.4   Card from computer-constructed punched card key.

entire area. Such cards and the equipment for making them has virtually disappeared since the first edition of this book was written. Nevertheless, workers in some parts of the world may still have access to suitable equipment, and since card keys have particular advantages, a brief account of them is retained here.

Computer-produced punched card keys are of the body-punched type. Although a computer makes them in the first place, they are used in the hand as before. An example of such a card is shown in Fig. 5.4, from a key corresponding to Barnett and Pankhurst (1974). The card can be printed in many different designs and colours, but generally has the columns numbered from 1 to 80. In this case the numbers are printed below row zero and at the bottom. The rows are identified as 0 to 9 by printing rows of digits across the card, except for the top two rows which are left blank. The top edge of the card is generally used for printing, and there is a standard coding scheme for combinations of holes punched in columns which correspond to letters, numbers, and punctuation signs. Using the 10 rows and 80 columns, there is space for 800 holes. Each card represents a character state, so that up to 800 taxa could be put in. In fact, the right-hand end of the card in Fig. 5.4 has been punched with holes which are codes for the character state and a card number, as printed in the top right margin, so in this particular example 44 columns have been used for taxa. The key from which this card comes covers 434 species of yeasts. The taxon which is represented by a punched hole is easily identified by its column and row number. For instance there is a hole in column 11, row 3, so this is species number 113 (*Candida steatolytica*). Because the columns of the standard computer card are numbered from one and not from zero, the list of taxa with their numbers begins with number 11, which is really the first taxon. In the example, the holes from column 46 onwards have nothing to do with the taxa; they are only there as a means of putting in the printing at the top correctly.

Keys can be punched onto computer cards by hand using card punching machines. This is tedious, inflexible, and prone to errors, so it is much better to use a computer to make the cards. Computer programs for making punched card keys have been described, e.g. Morse (1974), Pankhurst and Aitchison (1975a) and Shultz (1975). There is also a polyclave option in GENKEY (Payne, 1975). Sinnott (1982) has programmed a version where all the states of a character are on one card. The way these programs work is relatively straightforward. The data matrix has to be read in and then the computer has to go through each character and each state of each character. It then has to find which taxa show, or could show, each state and arrange to produce a card with holes in the right places. For variable characters several cards will need holes for the taxon concerned. For taxa with missing characters holes ought to be punched in cards for all states of the characters. Inapplicable characters do not need to have any holes punched for their states, since these will never be observed. The computer can also arrange to punch holes on the card for the character state and number. In the example (Fig. 5.4) the character is number 1 (cellobiose fermentation) and its state is also number 1 (+), and the card has been numbered 101. Similarly, state 3 of character 16 would be numbered 1603. The details of punching the cards depend on the type of computer used. The computer has to be able to punch cards with arbitrary patterns of holes on them, and not just the patterns which correspond to printable symbols.

The cards issue from the computer without any printing on them. Machines exist which can read the cards and print them automatically, a process which is called interpreting. The left-hand part of the card, which is meaningless for printing, is skipped over. There are also machines which can punch copies of packs of computer cards. The original computer can be used to make copies also. Hence the manufacture of any number of keys on punched cards can be an entirely mechanical process. If desired, differently coloured cards can be used in order to emphasise different kinds of characters. Alternatively, the cards can be coloured on the edges with felt pens.

Punched card keys have two great advantages: the user can choose any character, and can use the characters in any order. Nevertheless, they are still sensitive to errors for the same reasons as with a diagnostic key. In the past there was no simple and cheap method for creating and reproducing them, which must have restricted their application.

5.6 Matching methods

In this section a number of loosely related methods are described, all of which produce a numerical value by which identification is assessed. This value is produced by a comparison of the unknown specimen with all the taxa in the matrix and by selecting those taxa which give the best results. The necessary computations are generally impractical without the use of calculators or computers, which are now an essential part of the identification procedure. These methods require more effort on the part of the user than those described previously, and correspondingly give more precise and more reliable results, since they are all polythetic and do not demand that the data be without errors. There are, broadly speaking, two kinds of methods involving:

1) a measure of likeness between taxa, such as a similarity coefficient or a correlation coefficient. Included here, however, are Eucledian distance methods where distance or dissimilarity is calculated;

2) a measure of the probability of identification, such as those based on Bayes' theorem or by the use of discriminant analysis.

5.6.1 Simple matching

A simple similarity coefficient is defined below. The definition of similarities for identification can use the Gower coefficient (p. 54) with a little modification. There is a difference according to whether one taxon is being compared with another or whether a single specimen is being compared with a taxon. In the latter case one cannot necessarily expect a single specimen to show all the variation. This depends on whether the variation, if any, occurs within single organisms or between members of a population. As an example, suppose that a plant taxon can have leaves which are round or elliptic, depending on habitat. A specimen has round leaves. This agrees exactly with the taxon, if each individual plant is only expected to have one shape of leaf. If however, the taxon has round leaves at the base of the stem and elliptic leaves higher up, and the specimen has only round leaves, the agreement is not exact. For the purpose of comparing a specimen with a taxon in a computer program, the simplest course is to ignore the distinction between variation within and between specimens by assuming the former, and to calculate the agreement for a character as a fraction, namely

$$\frac{\text{no. of states shown in common}}{\text{total no. of states shown by both}}$$

This definition lends itself readily to computation because each state may be represented by a 'bit' in a computer word (see p. 130) and the ratio becomes

$$\frac{\text{no. of bits in the 'and' of the two characters}}{\text{no. of bits in the 'inclusive or'}}$$

Another question about agreement of characters concerns the significance of a negative match. If two taxa both lack a character of the presence or absence type, can one say that this is an agreement or should this be ignored? Practice varies on this point, but it seems more reasonable to allow negative matches when the organisms being compared are closely related, as is usually the case in identification by matching.

If desired, weights can be attached to the characters. The perceptron theorem (p. 10) is a proof that this can be done. Weights could be chosen subjectively to represent convenience or be calculated on the basis of the distribution of states (separation coefficient or information statistic). In order to give weights to the occurrence of rare states of characters, the weight could be calculated according to the particular specimen. This means that the weight given to a character is not fixed in advance, but is made small if the specimen shows a common state and large if it shows a rare one. If the data matrix includes a mixture of characters with different numbers of states, the many-state characters could be given a higher weight since they are each equivalent to several binary characters.

The question of weighting when applied to conditional characters causes difficulty. Suppose there is a presence-absence character which, if present, can have other characters depending on it. For example, consider the leaf of a plant which might have a margin which is entire (without teeth) or serrate (toothed). If teeth are present, they could have properties of shape, relative size, direction, and so on. A specimen with toothed leaves may be able to score agreement with half a dozen characters in all, whereas one with entire leaves will only score with one presence-absence character. This can be regarded as natural weighting, favouring specimens in their agreement with taxa which have a character present. Alternatively, the bias could be removed by giving a high weight to the controlling character for when it matches by being absent. The weight could be the sum of the weights of the dependent characters.

Finally, the similarity coefficient can be written in a more mathematical form, as

$$\frac{\sum_i w_i \, A_{ji}}{\sum_i w_i}$$

for the similarity between a specimen and taxon j, where w_i is the weight of character i, and A_{ji}, is the agreement between the specimen and taxon j for character i. Many other kinds of similarity coefficient have been proposed which could be used (Chapter 4 of Sneath and Sokal, 1973).

For completeness, the formula for the calculation of a correlation coefficient is given. If x and y are two quantitative variables, then the correlation between them, given N samples x_i and y_i, of each variable is:

$$\frac{\sum_{i=1}^{N} \sum_{j=1}^{N} (x_i - \bar{x})(y_i - \bar{y})}{\sqrt{\sum_{i=1}^{N} (x_i - \bar{x})^2 \cdot \sum_{i=1}^{N} (y_i - \bar{y})^2}}$$

where $\bar{x}$ is the mean of x and $\bar{y}$ the mean of y.

This is intended for N samples from two variables, whereas if x and y represent the states of characters of two taxa, each with N characters, the formula can still be used to calculate a number, but it will not have any statistical significance. This number can be calculated without difficulty if all the characters are quantitative continuous variables, but is harder to apply if some or all of the characters are qualitative. In the following account of identification by use of the similarity coefficient, one could use a correlation coefficient instead (see Gyllenberg and Niemelä, 1975).

Various programs exist for identification by matching with similarity coefficients, e.g. Pankhurst (1975), Ross (1975), Sneath(1979), Fortuner and Wong (1984), Fortuner (1986); and the MinIdent system of Smith and Leibovitz (1986) which is a matching program for identifying minerals. The example of output in Fig. 5.5 is from the former program relating to *Banisia*, a genus of tropical leaf moth (Whalley, 1976). The first line of the results is just a title or comment relating to the specimen, which is a male thought to be of species *fenestrifera*. There follows, among other things, a list of taxa which could be identified with the specimen. These are listed in sequence with the similarity as a percentage, the count of characters used and the taxon name. Only a

```
/BANISIA CF. FENESTRIFERA MALE
 SPECIAL CHARACTERS ARE -
     UNCUS/DIVISION
     GNATHUS/PRESENCE

  SEC    SIM.  COUNT             SPECIES

   1     91.6   53   *++         FENESTRIFERA
   2     78.3   25               INOPTATA
   3     71.3   52    ++         FURVA
   4     70.1   49   *++         INTONSA
   5     66.7   48    ++         IDALIALIS


 RESEMBLES GROUP    4

 SPECIAL TAXA COMPARED
    1    91.6 *                  FENESTRIFERA


REPORT ON TAXON    15
 CHARACTER STATE
      5      1
         DISTINGUISHED TAXA-    1    2    3    4    5    6    7    8    9
                               13   11   12   13   16   17   18   21   26
                               27   28   29   30   31   32   35

 27      1
     DISTINGUISHED TAXA-    2    11   23   25   27   31   32   35
```

Fig. 5.5   Example of output of program for matching by similarity (data by Whalley).

small proportion of all the taxa are listed, namely those which show the highest similarity. It is then the responsibility of the program user to choose the answer from the information provided.

The similarity values may not necessarily be very high percentages. One reason for this is the inherent variability of taxa, and the fact that a specimen will often show less variation than the complete taxon, so that when compared with it in a matching program, the maximum possible score is less than 100%. Experience suggests that a level of 60 to 90% is usual, with an error margin of about 5% depending on various causes discussed below. The count of the number of characters used is given because unusually low numbers of characters cause more error in the similarity, and a high similarity with a low character count ought to be treated with suspicion. For example, the second species in the list, INOPTATA, has a low count (25) but quite a high similarity. This comes about because this species is only known from a female, whereas our specimen was male.

The program provides various ways of helping to choose the final identification. As an option 'special' characters can be chosen. These are written out from the second line of Fig. 5.5 onwards, e.g. UNCUS DIVISION. The idea is that the specimen will present various obvious or prominent characters which are such that one would have difficulty, subjectively, in accepting an identity for the specimen which did not agree with most or all of these characters. The rows with plus signs before the species names signify which of these special characters agree. Plus stands for agreement and blank for disagreement. The special characters as named in the list from top to bottom correspond to the columns of plus signs from left to right. For example, the first taxon FENESTRIFERA agrees with both special characters but the second species agrees with neither. The more plus signs there are against the name of a species, the more reasonable this species would be as an identity for a specimen. The program also tries to assign the specimen to an intermediate taxon. Suppose the data matrix concerns a family of species, then the genera are intermediate taxa. The program finds the intermediate taxon which, on average, most resembles the specimen. Any species in the list which is a member of this intermediate taxon (e.g. genus) is marked by an asterisk, e.g. FENESTRIFERA, INTONSA, both in the same subgenus. Hence, one may take those names with an asterisk and the highest number of pluses as the most reasonable candidates. Notice that the word 'reasonable' was used, and not 'probable'. There have been no probabilities or statistical calculations involved, although the answer indicated above might in fact be the most likely one.

If the user of the program has some prior notion of which taxon the specimen belongs to, this can be specified as an option, shown further down under the heading 'SPECIAL TAXA'. The similarity data are printed again, as a precaution in case they did not appear in the list above. There then appears an account of the character states of the specimen which did not agree with the taxon, if any. In the example (Fig. 5.5), there were two such erroneous characters. Notice that the identification is still successful in spite of the presence of the errors. This information can be used to revise the description of the specimen or the definition of the taxon. There is also a warning that if the character state is added to the description of the taxon, useful distinctions between the taxon and various others may be lost. For example, in Fig. 5.5, character 5 for species 15 appears highly diagnostic.

While a program of this kind has some tolerance of errors, the results must still be checked by comparison with full descriptions, illustrations or preserved specimens. Ideally the correct taxon will appear at the head of the list, with the highest similarity, with all special characters agreeing and be assigned to the correct intermediate taxon. The margin of difference between the correct taxon and the next depends on the classification and the number of characters used. If in the classification taxa are grouped or clustered closely together, there will be few characters which differ between them. Also, if a large number of characters are used, this will increase the similarity when a high proportion of the characters agree. For example, if two taxa differ only by one character out of 50, they can at best only be separated by 2%. In this example errors could still be tolerated in the description of the specimen, provided that the critical distinguishing character was correct, since this would only reduce the level of similarity but not the difference. On the other hand, there is then the risk that some other taxon will appear more similar to the specimen than the right one, and come before it in the list. For a data matrix to give the best possible performance, it must contain at least one differing character for each pair of taxa, and preferably more. However, in adding a character to increase the difference between pairs of taxa which closely resemble each other, one is decreasing the proportional difference between other pairs which do not differ on this character. Hence, the most effective matrix, without regard to subjective qualities of characters, will be that which has the highest ratio,

$$\frac{\text{average no. of differing characters for pairs of taxa}}{\text{total number of characters}}$$

provided that all pairs of taxa are distinct. This is something which can be routinely checked during runs of identification programs, e.g. in key construction (Pankhurst, 1970).

For a variety of other ways in which the quality of a matrix can be checked, see the series of papers by Sneath(1979). These were applied to a special kind of data matrix with only binary characters. Various measures of character separation (Gyllenberg, 1963) were explored in order to find which were the best characters. Since good characters can be correlated, this is more useful for finding characters of poor information content. It is not necessarily a good idea to delete such poor characters because they may be vital for distinguishing particular pairs of species. Sneath explores the idea of the hypothetical mean organism, which is a fictional taxon exhibiting the commonest characters, and matches it with each of the real taxa. This gives a measure of the extent to which variability depresses the matching scores. Sneath also describes a way of finding out which are the most unusual characters for each taxon, based on an idea of Morse (1974), and remarks that this is useful for finding which are the poorly described taxa.

The above arguments assume that the data matrix is both correct and complete. The correctness of the data matrix can be ensured by careful compilation and checking, but the effect of missing characters is important. In the above account missing characters were simply ignored when calculating similarities. The result of this is that if the character had been known and had it agreed, the similarity would be correct but otherwise is in error by being too small. There is no way to overcome this difficulty except by making further observations to complete the original matrix. The benefits of doing this can be very marked (Pankhurst,1975).

The accuracy of the allocation of the specimen to an intermediate level taxon depends on the classification. The intermediate taxa must be genuine clusters, such that the average similarity between taxa within clusters is greater than that between clusters. The best way to ensure this is to carry out a numerical clustering on the same data matrix using the same type of similarity coefficient, and to choose the clusters from the results. Even so, if the taxa do not in fact possess the structure of clusters, e.g. when they exhibit a cline of variation, one cannot expect to be able to identify accurately intermediate-level taxa.

If the characters of the taxa are continuous quantitative, it is reasonable to represent the taxa geometrically as points in a multidimensional space. The states of the N characters are represented by the perpendicular distance of points to each of the N axes. One cannot picture this for N larger than 3, and in Fig. 5.6 only two dimensions are shown. The distance between two points in the diagram represents the dissimilarity between two taxa. The scale of each axis represents the weight of a character, so that if all characters are to have equal weighting, the scale on each axis should be the same, e.g. from zero to one. This method of calculating the dissimilarity between taxa is called the Euclidean distance method.

This approach is particularly suitable for describing what happens to specimens identified by a matching method which do not exactly fit defined taxa (Gyllenberg and Niemela, 1975). In Fig. 5.6 the variation of taxa is represented by the way in which points are clustered together. The centre of such a cluster is the typical example of the taxon, and can be found by averaging all the characters of all specimens which are believed to belong to it.

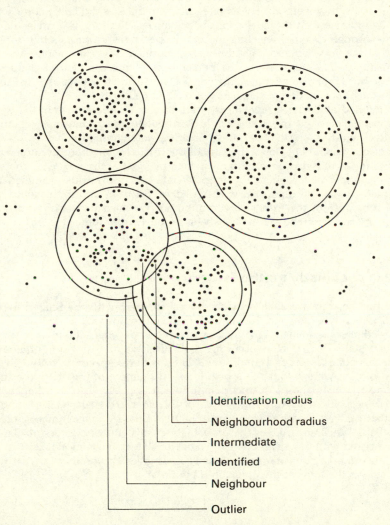

Fig. 5.6 An illustration of the four different identification states (after Gyllenberg).

If we draw a circle (in general a hypersphere) of suitable radius (identification radius) about the centre, we can decide that any specimen falling inside is correctly identified. We can draw a larger circle with the neighbourhood radius to cover specimens which are not near enough to the centre to be correctly identified, but which are still nearer to this taxon than any other and are neighbours. A specimen which falls outside either of these circles is an outlier and is not identified. We can also have the situation where two taxa are so close that their identification circles overlap, and any specimen which falls in the area common to both is an intermediate and cannot be assigned to either. It is clear from this how a computer would be programmed to identify specimens by this method. The choice of the radii is a difficult matter and depends ultimately on the quality of the initial classification. The circles must be large enough to avoid rejecting too many specimens as outliers but not so large that they overlap and have too many intermediates. An obvious way to choose the radii of the circles is by percentages of the commonest character states or by standard deviations. In practice, however, few data are available on the statistical variation of characters of biological species.

The method of Euclidean distances is an attractive one because of the way it can be pictured geometrically but unfortunately the characters for most biological identification problems are qualitative, not quantitative.

In passing it should be noted that any of the clustering methods of numerical classification could also be used as a means of identification. The unknown specimen would be added to the original data and the results examined to see which cluster the unknown is assigned to. Such an approach would be wasteful because of the extensive computations involved in working out the clusters afresh every time and has not been seriously used (but see p. 161).

5.6.2 Probabilistic methods

Under this heading we shall consider Bayes' theorem with the related maximum likelihood method and the method of linear discrimination.

Bayes' theorem is a means of making use of knowledge about how often particular states of characters occur for particular taxa and how often the taxa themselves occur, in order to find how likely it is that a specimen with a given pattern of characters belongs to a taxon. As an example of this, suppose that a rare taxon always has a character state which is rarely seen in other more common taxa. Evidently the occurrence of this character state makes it more likely that we have the rare taxon, but the rarity of the taxon itself makes it less likely. Bayes' theorem enables the probability of this situation to be calculated and compared with that of an unusual character state in a common taxon.

The theorem is given here without proof. It gives the probability that the specimen s is the same as the ith taxon (t_i) out of n

$$P(s = t_i) = \frac{P(t_i)\,P(s/t_i)}{\sum\limits_{i=1}^{n} P(t_i)\,P(s/t_i)}$$

where $P(t_i)$ is the probability of taxon i occurring, and $P(s/t_i)$ is the probability of s, given t_i, i.e. the probability that t_i has the character states shown by s. The probability $P(t_i)$ acts like a taxon weighting in this formula. $P(s/t_i)$ in turn needs to be calculated from the probabilities $P(c_j/t_i)$ that each character c_j in t_i has the right state, which is the product of all the probabilities of N individual characters multiplied together:

$$P(s/t_i) = \prod\limits_{j=1}^{N} P(c_j/t_i)$$

This is true provided that the characters c_j are independent of each other. If they are not, the proper approach is to find out by experiment what is the probability of occurrence of various combinations of character states which are known to depend on one another, but the number of possibilities to be accounted for may be very large.

The maximum likelihood method is closely related to this but gives all taxa the same probability of occurrence, i.e. $P(t_i)$ = constant, or equal weight to all taxa so that the formula reduces to

$$P(s = t_i) = \frac{P(s/t_i)}{\displaystyle\sum_{i=1}^{n} P(s/t_i)}$$

This simplification is often used not because the probabilities of occurrence of taxa really are all the same, but merely because they are unknown or variable.

Within the subject of biology applications of these methods are rare outside microbiology and agriculture, and it is worth giving the reasons for this. To begin with much laborious experimental work is needed in order to obtain the probabilities of states of characters. The probabilities of the occurrence of the taxa themselves are usually known in qualitative terms, e.g. common, rare. A more fundamental difficulty concerns the probabilities themselves; are they really probabilities? The definition of probability is the constant ratio of specific events to the number of samples taken. However, there are many situations where individuals of biological species have character states which are known to depend on the environment, according to the availability, for example, of moisture or food. Hence the proportions in which various character states occur within a taxon may be a function of other variables and not constant at all. It is also known that the genetic constitution of different populations of a species can be different, which can also result in varying proportions of character states between individuals in different places. Lastly, it is not always reasonable to suppose that specimens are sampled according to the proportion of variant individuals occurring in the wild (which itself can vary seasonally). The probability that particular species out of a genus occur will usually be very different in different habitats, and biologists themselves can greatly alter the probabilities by deliberately going to a locality where rare species are known to exist. For reasons such as these, Bayes' theorem or maximum likelihood is usually not applicable unless the sampling and the populations are carefully controlled, as for example with those bacteria which harm human beings or with varieties of crop plants. In situations where taxa overlap, however, a probabilistic method of some kind is a good way to distinguish taxa, and here Bayes' theorem or discriminant analysis is appropriate.

As examples of these methods, there are the programs of Baum and Lefkovitch (1972) for cultivars of oats, and Willcox et al. (1973) and Gyllenberg and Niemela (1975) for bacteria. Sneath (1979) describes a matching program which uses either Bayesian or similarity methods for identifying bacteria and also geological samples. The system described by Michalski and Chilausky (1980) for naming diseases of soybean crops is a matching program with weighted similarity coefficients, although it is presented as an expert system using probabilities. Payne (1975) has used Bayes' theorem to produce probabilistic diagnostic keys. The couplets where the taxa

```
FOR: ANYWHERE PHL                           OUR REF:9992/75 RUN V1
DATE: 24/04/75                                 (M619 LAB.1234)

YOUR REF: 123456        ATKINS, THOMAS

COMPUTER IDENTIFICATION BASED ON YOUR RESULTS, 28 TESTS DONE:

NOT IDENTIFIED, FURTHER TESTS SELECTED

YOUR RESULTS USED IN CALCULATION:


    MOTILITY 37    -   1    NITRATE         -   5    GLUCONATE      -   1
    GROWTH 37      +  99    SIMMONS CITR    +  85    MALONATE       -  40
    MACCONKEY      +  99    UREASE          -  50    ONPG           -   1
    CATALASE       +  99    GELATIN 1-5     -  25    GLUCOSE PWS    +  99
    OXIDASE        -   1    KCN             -  40    GAS GLUCOSE    -   1
    H&L OXID       +  99    H2S PAPER       -   1


    ADONITOL PWS   -   1    INOSITOL PWS    -   1    MANNITOL PWS   -   1
    ARABINOSE PWS  -  55    LACTOSE PWS     -   1    SUCROSE PWS    -   1
    DULCITOL PWS   -   1    MALTOSE PWS     -   1


    MR 37          -   1    VP 37           -   1    INDOLE         -   1


FURTHER TESTS SELECTED:

    FIRST SET                    SECOND SET
    ARGININE         9   1       TYROSINE PIG     8   5
    THORNLEYS ARG    9   1       CELLOBIOSE ASS   6  80
    INOSITOL ASS     4   1       GLYCEROL ASS     6   1
    TREHALOSE ASS    4   1       DULCITOL ASS     4   1
    SUCROSE ASS      3   1       FRUCTOSE ASS     3   1
    LYSINE           1   1       ETHANOL ASS      2  80
                                 PIGMENT          1   1
      SET VALUE =  30/ 30          SET VALUE =   30/ 30

DETAILS OF CALCULATION:

            GROUP                        SCORE
    ACINETOBACTER CALCOACETICUS        .963004
    PSEUDOMONAS CEPACIA                .020087
    PSEUDOMONAS PUTIDA                 .006919
    PSEUDOMONAS FLUORESCENS            .006362
    XANTHOMONAS SPP.(NOT HYACINTHI)    .002391
    PSEUDOMONAS FRAGI                  .000933
```

Fig. 5.7   Computer identification of bacteria by maximum likelihood method (after Willcox).

key out are labelled with the calculated probability of reaching that point in the key, and a threshold probability level is set to prevent couplets for very unlikely character combinations appearing.

   Some results from the program of Willcox are shown in Fig. 5.7 and these will be discussed in detail. This is a maximum likelihood method, which operates on a data matrix containing the probabilities of character states. These were established by careful experimental analysis of numerous examples (strains) of the different species included. Although some of the tests used are known to be (practically) always positive (or negative), the probabilities are never entered as exactly 0 or 1 but are approximated as 0.01 and 0.99, respectively. This is because a zero probability (for either positive or negative results) leads to a zero on the bottom line of the formula for maximum likelihood (p. 149) and the calculation fails. This situation cannot be ignored on the grounds that it has never happened so far because new results or observational errors can occur. The error introduced by this approximation is never more than one per cent in each probability value and is apparently tolerable.

The program proceeds by calculating the probability for each taxon, and then selects those which score most highly and, in this respect, resembles the similarity program described above. A score for each of the most likely taxa is printed at the bottom of Fig. 5.7. These scores are actually relative, not absolute, probabilities, since they have been multiplied throughout by a normalising constant so that they add up to one. The species at the head of the list, *Acinetobacter calcoaceticus*, has a score of 0.963, which looks impressive but is not in fact considered adequate for identification. The reason for this is partly that the real probability is not 96% but something different. Also, the criterion for identification used with this program is that the 'right' answer must have a relative probability of at least 99.9%. Put another way, this means that the summed relative scores of all the alternatives must be 0.001 or less, so that the score for the nearest contestant must be 0.001 or less. The actual probability will be different from this score but this will be ignored. Each good character which disagrees will give a factor of 0.01, because of the cut-off at 1%, so this means that a 'right' answer will agree by roughly one to two more characters than the nearest contestant. This could also only mean that the 'right' answer disagrees by a few less characters, most of the rest being totally wrong, so that as a check a list of aberrant results for tests is printed by the program for each species which is positively identified. In the example (Fig. 5.7), however, no definite identification is reached and so the program computes a list of further tests to be performed under the heading FURTHER TESTS SELECTED. The way in which this is done will be explained in a later section (p. 155). The program also gives, under the heading YOUR RESULTS. . ., the test results originally given (as + or −), together with the matrix entries expressed as percentages for the species with the highest score. It is interesting to estimate the similarity coefficient which corresponds to this situation. If every test result at 1% is regarded as a disagreement, there are 16 of these out of 28, so that the similarity is less than 50% even for the best answer. While identification in this particular program is by relative agreement, Gyllenberg and Niemelä (1975) show how an identification radius and a neighbour radius can be used with the maximum likelihood method.

Missing character state values in the data matrix cause a noticeable loss of accuracy for this method, just as they do for matching (p. 146). The Willcox program gets over this with the following strategy. First, the best possible situation, i.e. agreement, probability 0.99, is assumed for each occurrence of a missing value. If no definite identification is achieved with this optimistic assumption, the program just works out a set of further suggested tests. If there is a definite identification, the program repeats with the worst possible assumption, disagreement, for missing values. If after this, identification is still definite, identification is accepted. Otherwise the program works out a set of further tests as before.

A special problem occurs with conditional characters. An example of this for bacteria is growth and motility at 37°C (human body temperature). If a strain does not grow at 37°C, its motility will be negative. The result for motility is not just mostly negative if growth is negative; it is always so. The program has to anticipate and intercept this situation and substitute probabilities of nearly zero instead of zero exactly.

Discriminant analysis is another important statistical method which can be applied to identification, although it is strictly speaking a method for distinguishing between two or more populations. The identification problem is to distinguish one specimen from many taxa, which become analogous to populations if their variability is described. We have to regard the single unknown specimen as an approximation to a population. The basic idea of discriminant analysis is to find a boundary between two populations which is such that on the boundary a specimen is equally likely to belong to either population. In terms of Fig. 5.6, a line can be drawn somewhere between two identification circles so that character state combinations represented by points on the line are specimens which are equally likely to belong to either taxon or cluster. If we consider just two populations, which are both normally distributed with continuous characters and with the same covariance, an estimate of this covariance together with the two population means can be used to calculate a discriminant function of the form

$$y = \sum_i w_i C_i$$

where C_i is the ith character of the specimen, and w_i is a character weight, derived from the above calculation. If there are two populations, y is negative for one and positive for the other so that an unknown specimen can be assigned to one or the other by calculating y from its characters. This can easily be generalised to many populations (taxa) by calculating a y value for each population and assigning the unknown specimen to the population with the largest y. An explanation of the theory is given in Chapter 8 of Sneath and Sokal (1973).

In fact, most biological identification problems do not involve just continuously varying characters and even if they do, one may well not have normal distributions with equal covariance. In order to cope with discrete qualitative characters, where the normal distribution is not appropriate in any case, the distributions of the characters must be worked out in another way. This can be done by enumerating cases, which is laborious and requires much data. Alternatively, one can assume that the characters are independent and use the maximum likelihood formula to map the distributions, which is also laborious. These practical difficulties detract from what is otherwise a promising method in theory.

5.7 Matching keys

It is possible to combine some of the virtues of the diagnostic key with those of the matching method, in what may be called *matching keys*. A matching key may be presented in the same manner as a diagnostic key, or in the form of a table. This type of key was first applied by Evans *et al.* (1977). The following example is based on the *Epilobium* data matrix of Fig. 1.1

1 Score +1 for
   each of:
      Stem hairs appressed   Total score
      Stem with raised lines
      Stem without glandular hairs   more than -2: lead 2
      Stigma entire
      Calyx tube without glandular hairs

Score -1 for
each of
    Stem hairs spreading   less than -2: lead 3
    Stem terete
    Stem with glandular hairs
    Stigma lobed
    Calyx tube with glandular hairs

This is the first lead of a key which may continue with more similar leads, or with the regular type of leads as normally found in diagnostic keys. The user is asked to score points according to which states appear in the specimen. A plant whose stem is terete and has appressed hairs, without glandular hairs anywhere, and an entire stigma scores +3, and so the next lead to use is lead 2. Specimens do not necessarily have to agree exactly with either of the lists. It is possible to reach an ambiguous score, e.g. -2, so that both subsequent leads have to be explored, but this will not happen very often.

This kind of key can be set up starting with any *polythetic* classification, and it is not necessary for the classification to have been created by computer. All that is needed is a division of the taxa into two groups for each lead, so that the members of a group resemble each other more than the members of the other group. As a starting point, this might be the two subgenera of a classical genus. Suitable algorithmic methods are cluster analysis, ordination and reciprocal averaging, since these will divide the taxa into two groups at each stage. The method was first described by Hill *et al.* (1975) using reciprocal averaging (an ordination method).

Once the groups have been chosen, the *indicator value* for each state of each character is calculated, and averaged over the states for each character. The indicator value for a character state is defined as

$$\left| \frac{n1}{m1} - \frac{n2}{m2} \right|$$

where $n1$ taxa out of a total of $m1$ have the state in group 1, and similarly in group 2. This value will tend towards +1 when the character's states are different in the groups, and towards 0 when they occur equally often in either. If characters are constant throughout both groups, or if they are highly variable in both, they will have low values in either case, since they discriminate badly. It is not important whether the characters are binary or multistate, but it may be possible to get a higher value by reducing multistate characters to binary characters by recombining some of the states. Select a certain number C of characters with high scores. There is no ruling about how many characters to choose, or what indicator value level to stop at. However, the method will be more convenient and effective with C not too large and with high values. In the above example, C was 5 (out of 17 characters) and the lowest indicator value was 0.7. As above, for each group, tabulate the character states which are commonest. The highest and lowest possible scores are $+C$ and $-C$. Ideally, the members of one group will score from $-C$ to 0, and the other from 0 to $+C$. In practice, it is necessary to score each of the taxa in each group to find the range of scores. The boundary score is chosen half-way between the highest of one group and the lowest of the other, or if this is not possible, choose it in such a way as to minimise the number of taxa which do not fit. Taxa can score on the wrong side of the boundary because only C characters have been taken to approximate the differences between the groups, and C needs to be larger. It may not be possible to find a satisfactory group of indicator characters between two groups, and if so, this is a sign that the classification is weak. On the other hand, the groups may be so well distinguished by constant characters that leads in the style of a conventional diagnostic key are perfectly adequate.

Matching keys are particularly suitable for identification when the taxonomic groups are poorly differentiated (Gauld,1980), or where the groups are not separated by discontinuities, as is often the case in the classification of vegetation types (Evans *et al.*, 1977). They have the advantage that they are more accurate, especially when applied to poorly differentiated groups, but they have the disadvantage that more effort is required to use them. They can also be used when a natural (polythetic) key is required, but a natural key is likely to be harder to use and less accurate than the corresponding artificial key.

5.8 Character set minimisation

5.8.1 Definition of minimal sets

The question to be answered here is that of finding a way to make an identification with as few characters as possible. With diagnostic keys the key itself is a tentative answer because of the tendency to divide the taxa into equal groups at each stage, but with the matching methods discussed above it is better to have complete descriptions of specimens. If specimens are going to be described in full, we still want to avoid including characters which are not necessary. It is natural, then, to ask for the smallest set of characters which will separate all taxa, (the minimum character set). This need not be unique as there could be several minimal sets of equal size. In practice, the smallest set might be an impractical combination of characters, so that some other slightly larger set with more convenient characters might be preferred. In addition, the minimum set will very likely include only one differing character to distinguish some of the taxon pairs, and it might be better to ask for at least two distinguishing characters for each of the possible pairs of taxa.

The idea of a *diagnostic character set* or *diagnostic description* is closely related to the minimum character set. This is a set of characters which distinguishes a given taxon from all others. The question is, 'How do I know that I have taxon X, rather than any other?'. If the specimen agrees with every character in the diagnostic description of X, then that is what it must be. Diagnostic descriptions are often given in floras, monographs or handbooks and are mostly derived subjectively from experience.

The methods for finding minimum character sets and diagnostic character sets are very much the same, apart from the scale of the problem, so no distinction between them will be made in the discussion which follows. They are both examples of what is known as the *set covering problem*, which is famous for the difficulties it presents. This problem is an example of what is called an *NP-complete problem*. The meaning of this strange terminology is explained elsewhere (p. 83), but such problems have been proved to have no method for complete solutions other than an exhaustive search, which may be impossibly time consuming or expensive, even with a computer. Often the only alternative is to use a *heuristic* method, which aims at finding some sort of solution quickly, but has the disadvantages that there is no way to know whether the solution found is the best solution, or whether there are other solutions which are as good, and that the solutions which are found are no use as starting points for finding other solutions. Hence there are both exact and approximate methods for finding minimum character sets, and it may be necessary to compromise between speed and accuracy.

5.8.2 Exact methods

The exact method described below (Kautz, 1968) finds all sets of characters which distinguish all taxa, from which one can then choose the smallest or most convenient one. As a small example for the sake of illustration, take the first 5 taxa and the first 10 characters of *Epilobium* in Fig. 1.1. The table given below gives all characters which distinguish all the 10 possible pairs of species. The characters 1 to 10 have been lettered A to J. The rows and columns represent species numbers, so that in row 2, column 3, for example, the characters D(4) and G(7) distinguish species 2 and 3. Evidently there is no need to fill in row 3, column 2, as well because this would only repeat what is already known, nor the diagonals, which represent only the difference between a species and itself.

	1	2	3	4	5
1	–	HIJ	DGHIJ	CDEGHI	CEGHI
2		–	DG	DEGJ	EGJ
3			–	EJ	DEJ
4				–	D

There is no restriction in the nature of the characters which can be used, binary or multistate, discrete or continuous, constant or variable; the states only need to be non-overlapping. There is one catch, however, concerning conditional characters and variation. For example, character C(3) had different states for species 2 and 3, but it should not be put in the table. This is because character B(2) controls character C, and C can only be observed if B has state 'hairy'. Species 2 and 3 are both variable in character B, and so character C is not necessarily observable and cannot reliably be used to distinguish this species pair.

The table of differences can be much simplified. Compare entry 1-3 with 2-3. This shows that species 2 and 3 have characters D and G to distinguish them, and 1 and 3 have D, G, H, and J. Evidently D and G will be enough to keep both pairs separate, and so H and J are not needed under 1-3. We can therefore put DG under 1-3 instead. However, we already have this pair of characters under 2-3, so the entry under 1-3 can be removed altogether. This argument leads to the following rule: if any two entries are such that the characters in the shorter one are all included in the longer one, delete the longer one. The shorter set is said to 'absorb' the longer one. This also means that if any entries are identical with others in the table, cancel all but one of them. After these simplifications, the table reduces to:

	1	2	3	4	5
1	–	HIJ	–	–	CEGHI
2		–	–	–	–
3			–	EJ	–
4				–	D

We now have to find all the combinations of characters which will still keep all species apart. Let us begin by taking one character from each of entries 1-2, 3-4 and 4-5 and finding all the different combinations, 6 in all. These are easily seen to be:

HED, IED, JED, HJD, IJD and JJD

The last of these is the same as JD, since 'JJ' only means the same character twice over. Also, JD is included in JED, HJD and IJD, so these latter can be dropped. Putting these in order, we have:

DJ, DEH, DEI

Now combine these sets each in turn with the remaining one in the table, CEGHI. After simplification, there remain 7 sets of size 3:

CDJ, DEH, DEI, DEJ, DGJ, DHJ, DIJ

Character C is dependent on character B, so the first set is really BCDJ, and is not minimum size. BCDJ is called a minimal set, since although it is diagnostic, it is not of minimum size. The remaining 6 sets all involve only vegetative characters, and are acceptable.

This method can be carried out by pencil and paper, but even an example as small as that in Fig. 1.1. (13 taxa, 18 characters) is very laborious, and so the use of a computer is advisable (Willcox and Lapage, 1972). Even in a computer the amount of time and storage required increases rapidly with the size of the initial data matrix. The program described by Willcox and Lapage used only binary characters and only provided a minimum test set with a minimum of one distinguishing character for each taxon pair.

The Kautz method of combining sets has been generalised by Pankhurst (1983) into a method for finding diagnostic sets which finds all minimum and minimal sets over a given range of sizes and will ensure a given least number of distinguishing characters. Since the program is based on the DELTA format, all kinds of characters, binary or multistate, qualitative or quantitative, may be used. The only question that needs to be answered when comparing two taxa in a character is whether the taxa are distinct or not. Any kind of variation can be considered as long as overlapping states can be detected. There is one special case which is worth a mention, which is when dependent characters depend on a controlling character which varies, an example of this was given above (p. 30).

Suppose that diagnostic sets are wanted with a minimum of N distinguishing characters. The first task of the program is to compare one taxon with the others (for a diagnostic set for one taxon) or every taxon with every other (for the complete diagnostic set). This creates a table with a row for every comparison and with columns for characters (in which there is a 0 for when a character does not distinguish, or a 1 for when it does). This is the set of separating sets, and each row must have at least N 1's in it, or else there is insufficient data to give the minimum distinctions wanted. If there are any duplicate rows, these are discarded. If and only if $N=1$ any sets which are 'absorbed' can be cancelled as well, and then the sets are put in order of increasing size. The process of combining the separating sets now begins, starting with the smallest, and discarding duplicates and absorbed sets along the way. When all separating sets have been combined, only minimal sets will remain. The time for searching for absorption varies as the square of the number of sets, so absorption is checked for only occasionally. It is faster to just store the extra sets as long as there is enough memory space. This algorithm was still too slow, so a number of improvements were made.

Firstly, minimal sets can occur before the end of the process of combination, and they can be detected quite readily by looking to see whether the set shares at least N characters from each remaining separating set. Minimal sets do not need to be combined any further, but can simply be copied. This is because (without detailed explanation) they regenerate themselves and then absorb all the other sets they produce. This saves a great many operations. Secondly, the fact that a certain range of sizes of minimal sets has been asked for can be exploited. Once the first minimum set has been found, then the size of the largest minimal set is known (M, say), assuming that sets of all intermediate sizes actually occur. Combinations of sets greater than this size can then just be discarded, and this again saves a great deal of computation. Thirdly, there is a simple stopping rule, stated here without explanation. When all sets of size (M-1) are minimal, then all the required diagnostic sets have been found. Fourthly, once a minimum set has been found, it is possible under certain conditions (not detailed here) to skip many of the stages of combination of separating sets. Lastly, if memory space for sets runs out before the process stops, it is possible to take a risk by cancelling sets of the largest size (and give a warning message) and still obtain convergence in some cases. With all these improvements to the algorithm, a massive computation has been reduced to a large but feasible computation. The problem is still NP-complete; all that has been done is to find more efficient ways of carrying out an exhaustive search. In the examples given in the original paper, it proved practical to find diagnostic descriptions for species in a genus of 200.

5.8.3 Approximate methods

Approximate methods for finding a minimal character set, i.e. one which is reasonably small but not necessarily the smallest, may make use of a figure of merit for finding the best characters; for this the separation coefficient is very suitable since it directly measures the number of pairs of taxa which are separated. One method which has already been referred to is in the program for identifying bacteria by maximum likelihood (Willcox *et al.*, 1973) and is essentially that originally proposed by Gyllenberg (1963). When the identification score is inadequate, the program suggests further tests (characters) which ought to be carried out. It finds these by taking a selection of taxa from the list in order of the highest scores until the total combined score is sufficient (99.9 out of 100). Possible tests are those which have not already been used and which separate at least some pairs of taxa. To this purpose probabilities of test outcomes are approximated as positive or negative only. Tests are then selected in such a way that the next test taken is the one which separates the most additional pairs of taxa, while ignoring contributions to any pairs which are already separated by two or more tests. The addition of tests ceases when either all taxon pairs are separated by at least two tests or the available tests are exhausted. A similar program described by Rypka *et al.*, (1967) finds minimal test sets by calculating the separation coefficient for several tests at a time. To begin with the first test chosen is that with the highest separation. This first test is then combined with each of the remaining ones to make a test pair and the separation calculated for all these pairs. The pair of tests with the best separation is then combined with a third, and so on, until a complete set is found which separates all taxa. This method is a compromise between searching every possible combination, which would take an enormous amount of computer time, and simply selecting tests in the order of their separation, which would ignore important correlations between tests. Lastly, Payne *et al.* (1981) have programmed an approximate method in the form of a polyclave which can be used to select diagnostic characters.

The statistical methods of character-set reduction, discriminant analysis (p. 151) and principal coordinate analysis (Gower, 1966) are loosely appropriate for finding minimum character sets but do not actually guarantee that every taxon pair will be distinct. The character weights calculated by these methods are analogous to separation coefficients and indicate which characters are likely to be needed in a minimal set. Davies (1981) reports however that the separation coefficient and the information statistic are much superior to principal coordinates in this respect.

Another approximate method for finding good diagnostic characters was described above in the context of an on-line identification program (p. 122). A further method was described by Barnett and Pankhurst (1974). To find a diagnostic description for a given species, begin with the complete description of the species with all characters and then try removing characters one at a time. If the taxon remains distinct from all other taxa, that character can be dropped entirely; otherwise it must be retained. Different results will be produced according to the order in which characters are dropped. Hence, characters were tested for rejection in reverse order of their separation coefficient, worst first and best last. Care is needed with variable conditional characters, as described above, which may not always effect a separation.

Finally, Chvatal (1979), working in the context of non-linear programming, has published what is called the 'greedy' heuristic method. This can readily be understood by starting from the set of separating sets as described above, after the various simplifications have been completed. This set can be expressed as a table with a column for each character containing 0's and 1's. Each row of the table relates to a pair of taxa which may be distinguished by a character (marked with a 1) or not (marked 0). The problem is to find the minimum set, which is initially empty. Consider the column with the most 1's in it. This character is likely to be needed in the minimum set, so put it there, and cross out the rows which contain this character. Repeat this operation with the depleted table until all rows have gone. If the characters have a cost or weight, then when the 1's in the columns are counted, divide by the cost and take the column with the highest frequency to cost ratio. This method does not always succeed, but if it does it rapidly finds a single solution.

Lefkovitch (1985) has found an improvement to the greedy heuristic. He has shown that information theory can be applied to the minimum set problem to calculate a set of intrinsic costs which make the above algorithm perform better. He proposes a probability which can be calculated for each character which represents the chance that the character will be needed in the minimum set. This probability is obtained quite rapidly by matrix arithmetic. The starting matrix is the table as just described. Another matrix is obtained from it by putting 0 for every 1 and vice versa, transposing and multiplying the two matrices together, and the latent vector of the resulting matrix gives the probabilities. The cost of each character is then the negative logarithm of its probability, which is then used in the greedy heuristic as just described.

5.9 Continuous classification and identification

Since the matching methods of identification by computer use fairly complete descriptions of characters of specimens which are prepared for input to the computer, this provides an opportunity to refine the original database with the use of accumulated information on fresh material. This emphasises the fact that classification and identification are processes which form part of a repeating cycle. Roughly, the pattern of events is that, initially, a variety of organisms is collected and a classification is made from them, giving rise to keys or other means of identification. Subsequently, new material comes to light which cannot be identified satisfactorily, or new biological evidence comes to light, or both, and the classification has to be revised, giving rise to corrected identification procedures, and so on. This kind of cycle has been going on for centuries, but in some recent cases where computers have been involved the timescale has shrunk remarkably. This is particularly noticeable in the classification of bacteria which harm human beings, e.g. Rypka (1975), who coined the phrase *continuous classification and identification* to describe the cycle.

One cannot, however, simply take the description of a newly identified specimen and incorporate it into the original database without further ado. Assuming that the identification is correct, the specimen description needs to be checked in case any of the characters were wrongly observed. This is one reason why both the matching and maximum likelihood programs described above report on unusual character states in specimens which are positively identified. Even when unexpected character states have been checked, it may still be unwise to add all such new evidence to the database, unless sufficient cases of the new varieties have been observed. Otherwise, the tendency in the long run may be to obscure useful distinctions between taxa by accumulating records of rare and aberrant varieties.

5.10 Special techniques for identification

The background to this section has been given in Chapter 1 (p. 9). Any technique which gives rise to a reproducible graph on a data recorder or a consistent black and white pattern which can be digitised with a video camera might be suitable. Possibilities include chromatography in one or two dimensions, stained electrophoretic gel patterns, spectrophotometry, mass spectroscopy and neutron-activation analysis. Direct analysis of photographs is not promising unless the objects concerned are flat or symmetrical and simple in nature, e.g. insect wings, colonies of bacteria. More details are given in a review by Morse (1975). Another possibility is the analysis of interference patterns, applied to the recognition of diatoms (Cairns *et al.*, 1982). These methods show promise but are not yet ready for general use.

5.11 Comparison of methods

This section is intended as a guide in selecting a suitable method for an identification problem. No single method is suitable for all purposes. The simplest methods are the cheapest and easiest to operate and are also the least flexible and most error-prone. Conversely, the complex methods are more costly and complicated to use and are the most flexible and reliable. The simpler methods are adequate for small numbers of highly distinct taxa but something more sophisticated may be required when the taxa are numerous and closely alike. If the taxa overlap extensively, it is better to use populations and statistical methods. Little or no information is available regarding the

Table 5.1   Comparison of identification methods

	Diagnostic key	Punched card key	Matching		
			Similarity	Bayesian/ max. like.	On-line
Construction by computer	Yes or no	Yes or no	—	—	—
Needs a computer to use	No	No	Yes (batch) or no	Yes (batch)	Yes (on-line)
Can be used in the field	Yes	Yes	Yes or no	No	No
No. of characters needed per specimen	Few	Few	Many	Many	Variable
Works with fragmentary specimens	No	Yes	Yes	Yes	Yes
Result if some characters of specimen in error	Often wrong	Often wrong	Usually right	Usually right	Usually right
Can detect new taxon	Usually not	Usually not	Yes	Yes	Yes
Numerical estimate with answer	No	No	Yes	Yes	Yes

relative cost and effectiveness of the different methods applied to the same identification problem.

Table 5.1 compares the different methods on various criteria. The complexity of the methods increases from left to right, roughly speaking. A distinction is made between whether a computer is needed to set up the method on the one hand, or needed to operate it on the other. For those which can or must be operated by computer the usual mode of operation (batch or on-line) is given. Whether or not the method can be used in the field is shown next and this is just the opposite of the last criterion. The number of characters needed refers to whether the method is one of step-by-step elimination (monothetic) where relatively few characters are needed from each specimen, or whether it is one of comparison (polythetic) where it is better to describe the specimen completely. The on-line method can approach either extreme according to how it is used. Many biologists, such as palaeontologists or forensic scientists, are faced with fragmentary material where characters are missing at random, therefore need a multi-access identification method which allows them to use whichever characters are available. Curiously, the one method which is not suitable in these circumstances is the one which is currently the most popular - the diagnostic key. While the effect of errors has been discussed as appropriate under each particular method, the vulnerability of each method to errors of character description in specimens is much greater for monothetic methods than for polythetic ones. Only some of the methods give a numerical estimate of the correctness of the indicated identification, a consideration which is sometimes important. Correspondingly, those methods with a numerical estimate can show when the specimen is a member of some taxon other than those included. This error situation can pass undetected in step-by-step elimination methods.

5.12 Special kinds of specimen

Hybrids between species occur in nature and their identification presents difficulties. If a hybrid occurs frequently and has a characteristic appearance, it can be treated as a separate taxon and described like the rest. If many hybrids are possible in a taxonomic group, and if they are fertile and backcross further, the situation can be too difficult to cater for by adding extra taxa. A hybrid presented to a diagnostic key could then easily fail to key out, or could key out incorrectly. A matching procedure may do better because one or both of the parents can be expected to appear in the resulting list of taxa. This is because many hybrids are intermediate between the parents, or resemble one parent more closely than the other because of dominant and recessive genes. If there is such a degree of interbreeding that all kinds of intermediates occur, it may be necessary to lump both parents with the hybrids in one aggregate taxon in order to distinguish the whole from other related taxa. If the problem is only to distinguish a possible hybrid from its parents where all three may occur in the same locality, a *hybrid index* can be calculated. This is a similarity coefficient based on that set of characters in which the parent taxa differ. Clustering techniques can also be used to distinguish hybrids from their parents, e.g. Fitter (1980). This example involved 4 species of *Epilobium* and 3 hybrids between them. Representative specimens from the population are coded for the characters which are known to differ between the main species. A matrix of similarities is calculated and subjected to a clustering procedure and a dendrogram plotted. Specimens which represent the pure species will cluster together. The hybrids will appear in the same branch of the dendrogram as their parents, but further away from the centres of the species clusters. Adams (1982) compared various multivariate methods to test for hybridisation, and concluded that principal coordinates analysis was the most useful.

A similar difficulty occurs in medical diagnosis, but is not analogous to the hybrid in biology. This is *multiple pathology*, where the patient is suffering from two or more diseases simultaneously. The number of possible combinations is great, so it is not practical to describe them all. By and large all symptoms and signs (characters) of each disease occur, unless substantially the same parts of the body are involved, when they may interact or mask one another. The diagnosis has to account for all characters and this can be done by starting, fairly arbitrarily, with particular prominent characters and finding which diseases can account for these, until all characters are covered. One way to do this would be with a set of diagnostic keys, or equivalent, so that each key tackles a prominent character, e.g. fever, headache, and is cross-referenced to the other keys. Experience would still be needed in order to group the characters correctly. A large single key to all diseases would be much less helpful. Finally, there is the problem of mixtures. This is encountered by pharmacognosists who may be presented with a powdered drug which is an intimate mixture of products derived from several different plants and asked to name the constituents. There is not much that can be done in this situation apart from skilled guesswork, unless some of the characters seen in the mixture are uniquely diagnostic for particular plant products.

6

History of identification methods

This chapter is a brief outline of the history of the subject. Voss (1952) reviews it in more detail.

It is hard to say when mankind first began to classify plants and animals. The earliest 'folk' taxonomy was probably a very simple one with two taxa only: 'useful' and 'not useful'. Under 'useful' came anything which could provide food, medicine or shelter, and under 'not useful' came poisons, pests, weeds and everything else. Presumably recognition was by familiarity alone. The earliest written taxonomies were clearly hierarchical but there is no evidence that these were consciously used in the manner of keys. A typical passage from Aristotle, *Historia Animalium*, Book 1, Chapter 1, reads:

'Of land animals some are furnished with wings, such as birds and bees, and these are so furnished in different ways one from another; others are furnished with feet. Of the animals that are furnished with feet, some walk, some creep, and some wriggle.'

Theophrastus, pupil of Aristotle, prepared a detailed classification of plants and lists many binary characters. There followed a very long period of what, to modern eyes, seems to have been more or less complete stagnation in the study of natural history in the western world. Scholars were largely content to copy from older sources and to use their imagination rather than make observations of their own. Herbals and bestiaries of the middle ages were often illustrated in a fanciful way but must have been used to some extent for identification of specimens by comparison with the drawings.

In the 17th century a number of works appear where classifications are set out in diagrammatic form. One of the most striking is due to Morison (1672), discussed and illustrated by Walters (1975), as part of a classification of the *Umbelliferae*. Morison has drawn what is clearly a hierarchical tree (cf. Fig. 1.3) but does not state that it can serve as a key. Similarly Ray in Wilkins (1668) provides a table for familiar plants, and in the *Historia Piscium*(1686), published a 'table' of the cartilaginous fish (Fig. 6.1) both of which look just like keys, but again do not state that they are such. By contrast, Grew (1682) states quite clearly how to approach the writing of a key but does not actually carry out his own instructions. He comments on the need for a key and gives advice on choice of characters, as follows:

'Although many have bestowed extraordinary Care and Industry upon the searching out, and Description of Plants; and for the reducing of them to their several Tribes:

46   Lib. 3.

P i s c i u m

CARTILAGINEORUM

Tabula.

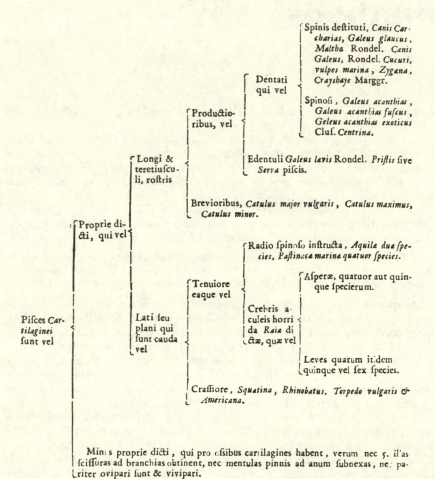

Pifces *Car-tilaginei* funt vel

Proprie di-
&i, qui vel

Longi &
teretiufcu-
li, roftris

Produ&io-
ribus, vel

Dentati
qui vel

Spinis deftituti, *Canis Car-charias, Galeus glaucus, Maltha* Rondel. *Canis Galeus,* Rondel. *Cucuri, vulpes marina, Zygæna, Crayshaye* Marggr.

Spinofi, *Galeus acanthias, Galeus acanthias fufcus, Geleus acanthias exoticus* Cluf. *Centrina.*

Edentuli *Galeus lævis* Rondel. *Priftis* five *Serra* pifcis.

Brevioribus, *Catulus major vulgaris, Catulus maximus, Catulus minor.*

Lati feu
plani qui
funt cauda
vel

Tenuiore
eaque vel

Radio fpinofo inftru&a, *Aquilæ duæ fpe-cies, Paftinacæ marinæ quatuor fpecies.*

Afperæ, quatuor aut quin-que fpecierum.

Crebris a-
culeis horri
da *Raiæ* di
&æ, quæ vel

Leves quarum itidem
quinque vel fex fpecies.

Craffiore, *Squatina, Rhinobatus, Torpedo vulgaris & Americana.*

Min¹s proprie di&i, qui pro ofsibus car¹ilagines habent, verum nec 5. il'as fciffuras ad branchias obtinent, nec mentulas pinnis ad anum fubnexas, ne. pa-riter ovipari funt & vivipari.

L I B.

Fig. 6.1   Table of the cartilaginous fishes (due to John Ray).

P R É L I M I N A I R E.   lxix

A N A L Y S E.

Fleurs dont les étamines & piftils peuvent aifément fe diftinguer.
1.

Fleurs dont les étamines & piftils font nuls, ou ne peuvent fe diftinguer.
16.

1.

Fleurs dont les étamines & piftils peuvent aifé-ment fe diftinguer...

Fleurettes nombreufes, réunies dans un calice com-mun.............. 2.

Fleurs libres & non réunies dans un calice commun.. 9

2.

Fleurettes nombreufes, réunies dans un calice commun.........

Fleurettes de même forte; elles font toutes en cornet, ou toutes en languette..... 3

Fleurettes de deux fortes, les unes en cornet, & les autres en languette..... 6

3.

Fleurettes de même forte...........

Fleurettes toutes en cornet............. 4

Fleurettes toutes en lan-guette............. 5

---

4.   Fleurettes toutes en cornet.

Carduus marianus.

---

5.   Fleurettes toutes en languette.

Hieracium murorum.

e iij

Fig. 6.2   Diagnostic key to higher plants (Lamarck).

yet I will take leave, here to propose a short Method whereby Learners, seeing a Plant they know not, may be informed to what Sort it belongs, and so be directed where to find it described and discoursed of For, except they have a Matter to conduct them, which few have; they must needs, by seeking at random, lose a great deal of time, which by a regular Enquiry might be saved. Besides, that which is learned by their own Observation, will abide much longer on their mind, than what they are only Poynted to, by another.

Now the most Philosophick way of distinguishing or sorting of Plants, were by the Characteristick Properties in all Parts, both Compounded, Constituents, and Contents. But of the Compounded, the Seeds and some other Parts, are oftentimes very minute: and the Roots always lie hid. As also the Constituent Parts, every where, without cuting and the use of Glasses. Nor can the Contents be accurately observed otherwise. So that for the Use here intended, those Properties are the fitest to be insisted upon, which are the most Conspicuous, and in those Parts, where the Learner may the most readily and without any difficulty take notice of them; as in the Flower and Leaf. The Flower hath varieties enough of it self. But in regard it is often wanting when the Green Leaf is not; it is therefore convenient, that he be assisted by both, and that the Varieties of both be distinctly reduced unto Tables. Which may be done, after the following, or some other like manner.'

[Here follows notes on the characters of plants. Then the final paragraph observes:]

'How far these, and some other like Distinctions, being reduced to Tables, would serve for the finding out of any Sort of Plant, may be conceived, if we consider, how great a Variety, a few Bells, in the ringing of Changes, will produce. And the search will be easy, and successful, if in every foregoing Table, reference be made to those that follow; and the Tables conteining the last Divisions, the Names of Plants therein poynted out, be expressed.'

Linnaeus, the 'father of modern taxonomy', described a key in 1736 and was the first to call it such (*clavis*, in Latin), but curiously his key was to botanists, not to plants! Nearly a full century passed after Grew's publication before the appearance of what are quite unmistakably keys, in the modern sense, in Lamarck's *Flore Françoise* (Flora of France) in 1778. Part of one of his keys is shown in Fig. 6.2. Lamarck describes how the keys are constructed and used, and understood their basic principles (cf. p. 92). In his own words (Vol. 1, introduction, p. lxxiii):

'Je dois observer ici que la manière de procèder dans une analyse ne peut être arbitraire, et qu'encore qu'il paroisse indifférent au premier coup-d'oeil d'employer telle division plutôt que telle autre, la marche, qui fera trouver le nom de la plante, doit cependent être combinée d'après certaines règles que je reduis à deux. La première est que l'on parvienne au but par la voie la plus sûre. La seconde est que cette voie soit en même-temps la plus courte possible.'

[I must remark here that the method of proceeding in an analysis (identification) cannot be arbitrary, and that although it may seem unimportant at first glance whether one division (character) rather than another is used, the path which will lead to the name of the plant has nevertheless to be constructed according to certain rules, which I reduce to two. The first is that one must arrive at the result by the most reliable route. The second is that this route should, at the same time, be the shortest possible one.]

In the two centuries since Lamarck, keys of various kinds have become the most popular means of specimen identification among biologists. A few additional ideas have been suggested in the meantime, such as keys with backward references (Bonnier, 1917), and the self-indexing variety due to Evans (1949) already referred to (p. 96); but the basic idea remains the same.

The 20th century has seen most of the innovations in identification methods. The idea of the tabular key, called by its author a 'synoptic key', appears with Ogden (1943) and Gyllenberg seems to have been the first to try out a matching type of program on a computer for a biological application (see Chapter 5). Cards for edge-punching were patented in the 1920s and the first applications to making keys appeared in the 1930s, e.g. Clarke (1937). The word 'polyclave' was first coined by Duke (1969) who used it for a card overlay scheme which is similar to the body-punched card key, for which the term is now often used. The first on-line identification program appears to have been that of Boughey *et al.* in 1968 (see Chapter 5). Monochrome graphics was first included in an identification program for fossils by Alexander (1985) and interactive colour graphics was introduced by Pankhurst (1988) with British orchids.

The application of computers to identification began in the early 1960s, some 10 to 15 years after the beginnings of computers themselves (usually dated as 1947) but quite soon after the appearance of general-purpose high level computer languages (late 1950s), which was probably a necessary prerequisite. It may well be true to say that most of the basic techniques for identification with the aid of a computer have now been worked out, and that we are now in a period of expansion of applications. The use of computers makes possible a very much wider range of different methods for different purposes and a much greater flexibility than the traditional techniques could offer.

7

Applications in computerised identification

This chapter will give some details of the kind of identification problems encountered in different branches of biology with some comment on medical diagnosis also, which is a rather similar problem. It is not intended as a guide to the principal works for the identification of the world's flora and fauna, although some such publications will be mentioned. Guides for this purpose already exist, e.g. Kerrich *et al.* (1978). Nor will it review the many techniques available for obtaining information about specimens, which range from direct observation to the use of complex laboratory procedures and large-scale electronic equipment; details of these are to be found in the appropriate standard taxonomic textbooks. Computer applications will be dealt with in their systematic context.

The following remarks apply to most taxonomic groups. The availability of means of identification varies according to the state of taxonomic knowledge of the group concerned. Where the taxonomy is in an early stage, there is a tendency for little to be available and that to be unreliable, e.g. for protozoa. Conversely, where taxonomy is more advanced, e.g. for higher plants in temperate regions, a wide variety of good keys are on hand. There are regional differences as well; for example, the temperate zones are far better studied than the tropical lowlands. Also, the degree to which different groups have been studied is related more to the ease with which they can be studied, their popular appeal and their economic or practical importance to man, rather than to their diversity or biological or ecological significance. The overwhelming majority of identification aids published are diagnostic keys of one form or another. The reasons for this must be their historical precedence, the practicality of keys in the field, and the ease with which they can be published and distributed. Recent technical innovations provide other ways of making identifications which are also practical in the field and are easily distributed, but which avoid the drawbacks of diagnostic keys, so this situation may be expected to change. Finally, it must be said that there occur instances in all parts of biology where there are numerous taxa to distinguish and although these may be all quite distinct, it is more effective to provide a good set of drawings or photographs than to describe the differences in words.

One difficulty which besets taxonomists of all kinds is the distortion or loss of information caused by the preservation of specimens. The problems include fading of colours, distortion of shape, lack of adequate field notes, and the loss or decay of soft or fragile parts. This is sometimes allowed for by providing keys which are especially intended for preserved specimens.

7.1 Botany

Botanists are generally well provided with keys, especially for vascular plants in temperate zones. There is less adequate provision for cryptogamic plants, the smaller fungi and tropical flora. There is a strong emphasis on mature (flowering or fruiting) material, and one would have much more difficulty in trying to name seeds, seedlings, or immature plants. Since both sexes usually occur on the same specimen, separate keys to male and female plants are not often needed. Computer-constructed diagnostic keys have begun to appear, e.g. Watson and Milne (1972) and Barnett and Pankhurst (1974). The monograph by Nooteboom (1975),on the genus *Symplocos* was the first to include computer constructed keys. The virtues of punched card keys have long been realised; centre-punched examples are the key to genera of tropical trees by Bianchi (1931), and the key to angiosperm families of Hansen and Rahn (1969). Other examples are the edge-punched key to eucalypts (Hall and Johnston, 1954) and a very extensive edge-punched key to wood samples (Phillips 1948), which is particularly intended for fragments. Examples of computer produced card keys include a key to mosses by Weber and Nelson (1972), and a key to grasses by Pankhurst and Allinson (1985), and the key to monocotyledonous families by Rao and Pankhurst (1986). The two latter keys also exist as on-line interactive identification programs. The key to Angiosperm families by Hansen and Rahn mentioned above exists as an interactive program (Duncan and Meacham, 1986), and this data has also been converted to DELTA format. The XPER program has been applied to tropical trees (Forget *et al*, 1986) and to mushrooms and toadstools (Lebbe, 1986). The latter system is remarkable in that it is available on-line to telephone subscribers throughout France. Tabular keys have already been quoted, such as those of Hedge and Lamond (1972), Tutin (1980), Sinker (1975) (p. 107) and Ogden (1943) (p. 167). Matching programs using similarity have also been discussed (p. 141), and there is a botanical example in Pankhurst (1975). The program described by Michalski and Chilausky (1980) for diseases of soybeans is a matching program with weighting. The derivation of the weights is supported by arguments from expert systems using probabilities. Palynologists have attempted to identify pollen grains in a similar way (Walker *et al.*, 1968). Baum and Lefkovitch (1972) applied the Bayesian method (p. 148). The original on-line identification program (Boughey *et al.*, 1968) was applied to the flora of Orange County, California. An expert on-line program with computerised images of the plant characters is available for the identification of British sedges (Pankhurst and Chater, 1989).

The types of vegetation in which plants occur can also be classified, and so there is an identification problem here too. The characters of the vegetation are the species which occur within it, and their relative frequency. It is possible to write diagnostic keys to vegetation types, e.g. Adam (1981). Matching keys are particularly suitable for recognising vegetation types (Evans *et al.*, 1977).

7.2 Zoology

It is said that three-quarters of the biological species in the world are insects. However, this is not to say that entomologists and entomological identification keys occur with the same relative abundance. Taking zoology generally, the diagnostic key is again the favourite method but zoologists are probably not so well provided for as botanists. It seems that the difficulties of making descriptions are greater and keys are frequently illustrated, e.g. Fig. 4.1. As a further example, the monumental, many-volume *Tierwelt Mitteleuropas* (Animal World of Central Europe) of Brohmer *et al.* (1960) contains numerous keys and illustrations. Quite often the standard reference works to animal groups simply contain illustrations and descriptions with few or no diagnostic keys, e.g. the FAO series on commercial fishery (1973) or one of the standard works on protozoa (Kudo, 1966). There is something of a tradition in some groups, e.g. butterflies moths, and birds, to have only volumes of descriptions and pictures and not to use keys at all. It may also be fair to say that zoologists (other than entomologists) have more difficulty in preserving specimens for study than do botanists. The need for different keys to males versus females, and larvae versus adults occurs frequently.

Entomological keys have been constructed by computers, e.g. Dallwitz (1974), and tabular keys have been put forward (Newell 1970). Gauld (1980) gives a matching key, which he calls a 'polyclade'. The program NEMAID described by Fortuner and Wong (1984) and Fortuner (1986) is a matching program applied to nematodes. The XPER interactive identification program has been applied to sandflies by Lebbe *et al.* (1987), and PANKEY to beetles (von Hayek, 1990). Examples of the use of discriminant analysis in zoology are given by Sneath and Sokal (1973). It seems that as yet there are not as many examples of zoological identification by computer as there are in other disciplines.

7.3 Palaeontology

This subject presents some contrast to botany and zoology. The palaeontologist is frequently faced with fragmentary specimens, especially of larger vertebrates. There is also the effect of accidents of preservation, where specimens are crushed or distorted, and where some of the characters which appear to be present really derive from the rock rather than from the original organism. The general custom is to compare specimens with collections or illustrations rather than to use keys. There are a number of impressive general publications which are well illustrated, but which contain few or no keys, such as the many-volume *Treatise on Invertebrate Palaeontology* (Geological Society of America), and the catalogues for the Foraminifera (Ellis and Messina, 1940), and for the Ostracoda (Sylvester-Bradley and Siveter, 1973), where the illustrations are photographs in stereo pairs. There are exceptions to this general rule, such as the keys to fossil corals (Cotton, 1973) and in palaeobotany (Harris *et al.*, 1961).

If the reasons for the unpopularity of diagnostic keys in this area is the problem of fragmentary specimens, there is much scope here for the application of the other methods. The only computer application known at this time is a database on fossil pollen grains (Germeraad and Muller, 1972). In this case, nonetheless, specimens are generally complete, if distorted. This data base is used for identification by searching via information retrieval techniques, which is a form of matching by similarity.

7.4 Microbiology

Microbiologists can preserve their specimens as can other taxonomists but they cannot 'see' their specimens in the same way since the characters are not self-evident as they are, say, on a herbarium sheet or in a spirit jar. The characters are mostly chemical tests, taking a long time to complete, and so the results usually get coded onto record sheets. There are few or no morphological characters. Given the amount of identification work in bacteria which is carried out at public health laboratories, large amounts of descriptive specimen data accumulate quickly. These are probably the reasons why bacteriologists began to use computer methods before other taxonomists, both in classification and identification.

Because the tests take a long time, they are carried out in batches. If identification is attempted with a diagnostic key, and a character (test) which is requested has not been done, one is in much the same situation as any other biologist with a fragmentary specimen. If the specimen comes from someone who is ill in hospital, there may not be time for more tests to be completed to establish the identification before treatment can begin. On the other hand, the tests cost money and it is not reasonable to carry out all tests on all specimens. In addition, bacteria often occur in typical 'strains' as a result of relatively rapid evolution, and for all these reasons multi-access or polythetic identification methods seem to be preferred.

Conventional diagnostic keys for bacteria seem to be few but there have been many computer applications. Punched card keys have been prepared and one, the Pathotec Rapid Identifier produced by General Diagnostics Inc. in 1975, is commercially available. A mechanical polyclave for bacteria (Olds, 1970) was described on p. 104. In the class of matching methods, the work of Gyllenberg (1963) and Gyllenberg and Niemela (1975) has been discussed (p. 146), and the program of Willcox et al. (1973) has been described in detail (p. 150). These methods often use the maximum likelihood approach because of the availability of data on the probability of the occurrence of character states. A considerable number of related papers have appeared since 1970 (see the review by Willcox et al., 1980)

There has also been some work on yeasts which are very useful in brewing and food manufacture. Barnett and Pankhurst (1974) have a lengthy computer-constructed diagnostic key, for which an equivalent punched card key exists and a set of computer-derived diagnostic descriptions. A matching procedure for computer identification of yeasts is described by Campbell (1973). More recently, Barnett, Payne and Yarrow (1985) and Esterre, Vignes and Lebbe (1987) have described on-line programs for yeast identification.

7.5 Pharmacognosy

Pharmacognosy is the study of natural products (mostly from plants) giving rise to pharmaceutical products. Pharmacognosists are often asked to identify the raw materials of drugs, usually powdered plant material, root segments or fruit. When the material is a mixture the identification problem is severe (p. 162). There exist illustrated textbooks showing the microscopic details of such materials, e.g. starch grain type, oxalate crystal shape. One difficulty is the unrestricted variety of plant products which may be encountered, so that it is hard to make a key complete. There is, however, one large diagnostic key (Claus, 1956) and a punched card key (Nelson, 1972). Ritchie *et al.* (1975) describe a punched card key aimed at recognising drug tablets from their external appearance for use in cases of drug abuse. Jolliffe and Jolliffe (1976) describe a computer program for identifying drug materials which uses matching by similarity.

7.6 Medical diagnosis

Medical diagnosis is not, of course, a biological problem except in the widest sense, but it is very interesting to compare it with biological identification.

A disease is not strictly analogous to a biological taxon because there is not a similar body of theory to explain why it is separate from other diseases and how it maintains this separation. On the other hand diseases are in fact largely distinct from each other; if they were not, there could be no diagnosis. Whether a disease is something which exists in its own right, or whether it is simply a convenient label for the correspondence between a set of symptoms and a course of treatment, is not a question which has to be answered before diagnosis and treatment can be carried out. However, many diseases have known causes, such as infection by bacteria or some bodily malfunction, which can often explain the symptoms. In fact the 'characters' of a disease are of three kinds: (i) symptoms, which the patient is aware of and may complain of; (ii) signs, which the doctor observes but which the patient may not know about; and (iii) tests, often chemical and quantitative, usually carried out in a laboratory on a sample. These distinctions do not affect the logic of diagnosis but tests tend to be more expensive or inconvenient for the patient.

Human diseases are very few in number (thousands) compared with biological species (millions). A naive and ignorant biologist might expect to find that these diseases were all thoroughly classified and described in textbooks of medicine, along with suitable keys for recognising them. Certainly there are medical textbooks which describe diseases but their classification, compared with biological classifications, is rather unfinished. There are good reasons for this; one is that taxonomic studies are not the most urgent priority for the medical profession; another that diseases are quite high-level taxa, corresponding, say, to the level of the family rather than the species, and include a great deal of variation. While the development of a disease from its beginning to its climax corresponds to the changes in an organism from birth to maturity, there is nothing biological which really corresponds to the variation in disease characters brought about by different stages in different possible courses of treatment.

Doctors mostly seem to be taught to diagnose by looking at examples rather than by following an explicit logical procedure. In a survey, Freemon (1972) found that more than half the medical staff questioned thought that they diagnosed by some kind of step-by-step elimination of diseases by characters, whereas others thought that they did some sort of matching or assessed probabilities of different diseases. There certainly exist diagnostic characters which are specific, or nearly so, to particular diseases, e.g. the spasm of the jaw muscles seen in tetanus, but only some diseases can be recognised by such means. There is, therefore, more or less nothing in the conventional practice of medical diagnosis to correspond to the use of diagnostic keys by biologists.

The first applications of computers to medical diagnosis appeared at about the same time as biologists began to apply computers to identification problems. An important instance is the program of Brodman *et al.* (1959) which was a form of matching by similarity with character weighting. Most of the programs since then have employed Bayes' theorem of maximum likelihood, as described in the review by Croft (1972), where a plea is made for a concerted effort to compile a definitive set of standardised disease descriptions, which scarcely yet exists, and for study of the comparative effectiveness of different methods. A biologist might be surprised to learn that the diagnostic key and the punched card key, or other forms of polyclave or tabular keys have scarcely been tried in medical diagnosis. Notable exceptions are the logoscope (Nash, 1960) (see p. 108 and Fig. 4.7) and the diagnostic flowcharts of Essex (1975). The diagnostic flowcharts are logically the same as diagnostic keys, except that they are drawn in the form of decision trees, as the key in Fig. 1.3, with the questions (characters) in boxes joined to other boxes by arrows. These charts were prepared for use in rural communities in Tanzania and were given field trials to ensure accuracy. The use of many different flowcharts, each for a prominent symptom or symptom group with cross-references, is a solution to the problem of multiple pathologies referred to earlier (p. 162). Hence one may say that all the various methods have yet to be fully tried out in medical diagnosis, as is also true in biology but the pattern of use and development has so far been very different.

7.7 Miscellaneous

One key which does not fit into the above categories, but which obviously serves a popular demand is the key by Dussart (1980) for choosing which statistical tests can be used for different kinds of data analysis. The MinIdent program for the identification of minerals (Smith and Leibowitz, 1986) is a kind of matching program. Sneath (1979) also gives a geological example.

7.8 Summary

The previous discussion has not covered every possible area of application for identification techniques in biology but an effort has been made to cover all the kinds of problem which can occur. In the author's view, both the problems and their solutions are more uniform than is generally supposed to be the case.

8

Expert systems

8.1 Introduction

Expert systems is the name given to a body of techniques in computer science which are intended to solve a certain class of problems. It is currently difficult to find very many examples of expert programs (in the official sense) being applied in taxonomy. Hence this chapter will differ from earlier chapters, in that the discussion will concentrate more on an explanation of the techniques than on their applications. In addition, it will be argued that some of the potential applications of official expert systems to taxonomy, as in identification, are already covered by existing methods.

An expert system may be defined in various ways, but the simplest definition is to say that it is a computer system which performs functions which are similar to those normally performed by a human expert (Goodall, 1985). Various qualifications should be added to this, namely:

1) that the computer system uses stored knowledge, in some suitable form. This is often known as the *knowledge base*.

2) that the computer system applies some reasoning mechanism to this knowledge, in order to prompt or take decisions. This control system is often called the *inference engine*.

Three more points may be made, which are not necessarily part of the definition, namely:

3) that the expert system may handle uncertainty,

4) that it may be able to provide some explanation of its reasoning, and

5) that it should be able to adapt itself progressively to shortage of information. To put this another way, the system should not fail totally and immediately if it should happen that one or more data items are unavailable, but instead it should try to use other data, or else it should attach more uncertainty to any conclusions that are offered. Behaviour of this kind is known as *graceful degradation*.

There are two general areas to which expert systems might be applied in taxonomy. These are identification (see Chapter 5) and interpretation (advice-giving), by which is meant the application of a published rule book or official regulations to making a decision. For example, an expert system might conceivably be used to help decide whether or not the publication of a taxon is valid according to the rules of botanical, zoological or bacteriological nomenclature. ESP Advisor (Anon, 1985) is a program which would be suitable for this.

It often happens with commercial or industrial applications of expert systems that it is desirable to model the behaviour of human experts. To do this, the expert is interviewed by a computer scientist in order to establish and code the knowledge base. Surprisingly, it is often found that the expert may be unable to express his or her knowledge or skills in the necessary form without outside help. The process of creating the knowledge base is known as *knowledge engineering*.

Alternatively, if a set of solutions to a problem is available, expressed as named items with their properties described, then it is possible to write a program to construct decision trees, i.e. a set of rules. This has been called *rule induction* (Quinlan, 1979 and 1985). Quinlan used a measure based on information statistics in order to decide between properties. The use of expert system terminology in these publications obscures the fact that these are really key construction programs, closely analogous to the earlier programs produced by taxonomists viz. Dallwitz (1974), Hall (1973), Morse (1974), Pankhurst (1970 and 1971), Payne (1975), and Ross (1975). The analogy is particularly strong for Dallwitz's program where the information statistic is also used.

8.2 Knowledge representation

There are currently a considerable number of ways to represent knowledge, each of which is particularly suitable for one or more applications. A scheme commonly used in computer science is what is called a *production rule*. As an example consider:

> IF the stems are hairy
> AND the flowers are rose pink
> THEN it is *Epilobium hirsutum*

These are just two diagnostic characters, or a diagnostic description, as taxonomists have been long accustomed to use. The rule is simply based on the *fact* that there exists something called *E. hirsutum* which has these two characters. More formally, this is a statement in what is called *propositional logic*, also known as Boolean logic. In other words, it is a series of facts connected by the operators 'and' and 'or'. In fact, this rule as just stated is not strictly accurate, since there are other *Epilobium* species with hairy stems and rose pink flowers, and there are other plants which have hairy stems and rose pink flowers which are not a species of *Epilobium*. To allow for this, the rule could also have uncertainty or a probability attached to it, so that the last line of the example could read

> THEN it might be *E. hirsutum*, or
> THEN it is 20% likely to be *E. hirsutum*

The final phrase could also be an instruction or an action rather than a statement, as in the following description of the Death Cap:

> IF the toadstool has a greenish cap
> AND it has white gills
> AND it has a sheath round the base of the stem
> AND is growing under oak trees
> THEN don't eat it!

It is immediately obvious that these rules closely resemble the leads of a diagnostic key, with the very important difference that these rules are the *data* for the method, and not the *output* key (or set of rules) produced by one of the various key-constructing methods!

A suitable data structure for storing a scheme of rules in computer memory is a *list structure*. There is a computer language called LISP which is designed to manipulate just such a data structure. An explanation of the relevance of LISP to expert systems is given in Goodall (1985).

Another way of representing rules is by means of what is called *predicate logic*. This is a formal means of stating the properties of objects and the relationships between them. Statements could be made about the properties of an unknown specimen called 'myplant' such as

stem_type(myplant,hairy).
petal_colour(myplant,rose_ pink).

and the definition of '*E. hirsutum*' could be

E_hirsutum(X):-stem_type (X,hairy),petal_colour (X,rose_ pink).

which is to be read as 'IF X has hairy stems AND rose pink petals THEN X is *E. hirsutum*', just as above. A programming language called PROLOG (see, for example, Burnham and Hall, 1985) has been designed in order to make statements like these and to make deductions from them. PROLOG is distinctive in that it is a non-procedural language. That is to say that there is nothing in the language which states how a problem is to be solved, but only the means to state the facts and to pose the problem. In order to ask in PROLOG whether my plant is *E. hirsutum*, the statement would be

?E_hirsutum(myplant).

It is evident that the examples of facts expressed above in PROLOG are analogous to taxonomic descriptions in the DELTA format. A statement such as

stem_type(taxon,hairy).

is just a character and state data matrix entry for 'taxon'. Similarly, the above definition of *E. hirsutum* is equivalent to an extract from a column of the data matrix. There is also a close analogy between the data statements of PROLOG and the records of a database system, where the characters would be the fields of records which represent taxa.

Other data structures which have been used for representation of knowledge include graphs, semantic networks, and frames. A graph in the mathematical sense is a series of points joined by lines, but without there being any closed internal loops. The points represent the objects and the lines between them represent the relationships. This is illustrated by the minimum spanning tree, Fig. 3.7. A semantic net is similar, but loops are allowed. A frame consists of blocks of data of different sizes which are connected by pointers. The diagram of a database field and record structure in Fig. 2.2 is rather like a set of frames. The data matrix (p. 2), which is the basis of so many programs which handle descriptive taxonomic data, does not seem to have been much favoured for expert systems, although it is possible that Expert Ease (Anon, 1983) uses it. For more details of data structures for expert systems, see Hayes-Roth *et al.* (1983).

8.3 Deductions from knowledge

By far the commonest approach to representing knowledge in expert systems is via rules, and thereafter the usual method for making deductions from rules is to search trees for rules or combinations of rules which satisfy the questions. This is likely to be the way that a PROLOG question like that just given would be resolved.

Two strategies for making deductions are current in expert systems, namely:

1)   the *forward-chaining* or *data-driven* strategy, which starts with the data and attempts to see what conclusions can be drawn from it,

2)   the *backward-chaining* or *goal-driven* strategy, which starts with a goal (assumption, hypothesis) and tries to confirm this with the available data.

An example of forward-chaining is found in the conventional use of a diagnostic key, starting with the first lead, and working forward (or down) its logical tree structure. The same key might also (with more difficulty) be used backwards, by assuming the name of the taxon to which the specimen belongs and starting where it keys out and trying to find a path back up to the first lead. This is a kind of backward chaining. This analogy with diagnostic keys is an oversimplification; many expert systems allow for more than one alternative rule to be considered at any one time, and offer some means of deciding which rule to use, i.e. they allow multi-access. This is like having a choice among several leads, instead of just a choice of the questions within one lead. In interactive identification programs (p. 117) the data-directed strategy corresponds to commands like the BEST command, and the goal-directed strategy corresponds to the DIAG command, which attempts to diagnose a particular taxon.

In many situations a human expert shows the ability to work with incomplete or uncertain data. In a decision process there are a lot of "maybe" and "don't know" answers to the expert's questions, and still he or she is often able to reach some conclusion. In biological taxonomy this is also true, but when computers are applied to taxonomy it often turns out that data matrices can be defined with a reasonable level of precision without probabilities, when it is not possible to obtain the necessary frequency data. Most of the biological examples where uncertainty is used are applications involving microbes. There are today several techniques or theories of how to represent *reasoning with uncertainty*, and among the most usual are:

1)   Bayes' theorem (see p. 148). This has the disadvantage that the variables (characters) are assumed to be independent, which is normally untrue.

2)   MYCIN model of uncertainty (Gordon and Shortliffe, 1985). MYCIN (Shortliffe, 1976) is an expert system for the diagnosis of bacterial infections.

3)   Demster-Shafer theory of evidence (Shafer, 1976; see also Atkinson and Gammerman, 1987)

4)   Fuzzy logic (Mamdani and Efstathiou, 1985).

8.4 Applications in taxonomy

What might be called the 'official' expert systems began to be publicised at about the beginning of the 1980s, whereas the first advances in taxonomic computing were made about a decade before that. Consequently, there are rather few examples available of expert systems which have been applied to taxonomy, and the distinction between the expert systems approach and the taxonomic computing approach is not always clear. All the known examples actually apply to identification procedures. The identification programs are mostly of the interactive kind, but there are a few programs for key construction as well (Quinlan, 1979 and 1985). No applications of advice-giving programs are known. Some striking differences are apparent:

1)   The natural data format for taxonomy is the data matrix, whereas the natural knowledge representation or data input for expert systems is a set of rules. In fact, not a few of the taxonomic programs (for key construction, and for finding diagnostic descriptions) produce sets of rules as their *output*, and these are regarded as the finished product. The reason for this fundamental difference is probably that the expert system formulation is a generalisation for a wide class of ill-defined problem situations. In taxonomy on the other hand, both the data and the methods of solution are usually well-defined, or if not, can be made so.

2)   Taxonomic systems rarely include a control system, and users are deliberately left free to choose their own strategies for identification. It is evidently felt that a control system would be an imposition on taxonomist users.

3)   Data about probabilities of characters and taxa and the need to handle probabilities are uncommon in taxonomy, and uncertainty can be dealt with in other ways, as by the use of the variability limit (p. 122).

On the other hand, it is clear that some of the important features of expert systems are shared by their taxonomic counterparts, such as the explanatory capability, and graceful degradation (see p. 123). It might be said that the taxonomic identification programs take advantage of the data matrix as a special case of knowledge representation and function internally in a quite different fashion, but externally have very much the appearance of expert systems.

Some brief notes on published expert systems will now be given. In spite of its name and the fact that it was marketed as an expert system, XPER (Lebbe, 1984) is very much a taxonomic system. It was written in BASIC and uses a data matrix, and has been applied to tropical trees, sandflies, yeasts and toadstools. Thompson and Thompson (1985) provide a readable explanation of how an expert system might be applied to the identification of plants, and they describe the plants using rules. In a general discussion of expert systems for entomology, Stone *et al.* (1986) mention a program called SYSTEX which was applied to the identification of the genus *Signiphora* (Hymenoptera). Thonnat and Gandelin (1988) describe an interesting system which goes the whole way from analysing two-dimensional images containing a rather diverse selection of species of zooplankton to the identification of the organisms present. It would be interesting to see whether their method would work with a selection of closely related and rather similar organisms. The FOSSIL system (Alexander, 1985 and Brough and Alexander, 1986) is a proper expert system for identifying fossils, using rules and PROLOG. It was also the first identification program to make use of (monochrome) graphics. Michalski and Chilausky (1980) describe a system for identifying diseases of soybeans, which gives an interesting account of a scheme for weighting characters, but in spite of its expert system context, it might just as well be described as a matching program (p. 141). Atkinson and Gammerman (1987) describe an expert program for identification which uses the Demster-Shafer theory of evidence to handle uncertainty, which they claim makes the system easier for non-expert users. Their data relates to flowering plants (Umbelliferae in Britain).

References

Abbott L A, Bisby F A and Rogers D J, 1985: *Taxonomic analysis in biology*. Columbia University Press, New York.

Adam P, 1981: The vegetation of British saltmarshes. *New Phytologist*, **88**, 143–196.

Adams E N, 1972: Consensus techniques and the comparison of taxonomic trees. *Systematic Zoology*, **21**, 390–397.

Adams R P, 1982: A comparison of multivariate methods for the detection of hybridisation. *Taxon*, **31**, 646–661.

Adey M E, Allkin R, Bisby F A, White R J and MacFarlane T D, 1984: The Vicieae database: an experimental taxonomic monograph. In *Databases in Systematics*, Allkin R and Bisby F A, (eds) 175–188, Academic Press, London and Orlando.

Alexander I F, 1985: FOSSIL: an expert system for palaeontology. *Tertiary Research*, **7**, 1–11.

Allkin R and Winfield P J, 1989: *ALICE User Manual*. (Version 2). Royal Botanic Gardens, Kew, England.

Anderberg M R, 1973: *Cluster Analysis for Applications*. Academic Press, London and Orlando.

Anderegg D E, 1989: *TAXADAT User's Manual*. University of Idaho, Moscow, USA.

Andre H M, 1988: Age-dependent evolution: from theory to practice. In *Ontogeny and Systematics*, Humphries C J, (ed.), 137–187, Columbia University Press, New York.

Anon, 1984: *Expert Ease User Manual*. Intelligent Terminals Ltd., Glasgow.

Anon, 1985: *ESP Advisor: user guide and reference manual*. (Issue 2). Expert Systems International Ltd., Oxford.

Anzovin S, 1988: *Quick and Easy Guide to HyperCard*. Compute! Publications Inc., Greensboro, N. Carolina.

Atkinson W D and Gammerman A, 1987: An application of expert systems technology to biological identification. *Taxon*, **36**, 705–714.

Babaç M T and Bisby F A, 1984: A chemotaxonomic database. In *Databases in Systematics*, Allkin R and Bisby F A, (eds) 209–218, Academic Press, London and Orlando.

Barnett J A and Pankhurst R J, 1974: *A new key to the Yeasts*, North Holland, Amsterdam.

Barnett J A, Bascomb S and Gower J C, 1975: A maximal predictive classification of a Klebsielleae and of the yeasts. *Journal of a General Microbiology*, **86**, 93–102.

Barnett J A, Payne R W and Yarrow D, 1985: *Yeast Identification Program*. Cambridge University Press, Cambridge and London.

Baum B R, 1984: Application of compatibility and parsimony methods at the infraspecific, specific and generic levels in Poaceae. In *Cladistics: perspectives on the reconstruction of evolutionary history*, Duncan T and Stuessy T F, (eds), 192–220, Columbia University Press, New York.

Baum B R and Lefkovitch L P, 1972: A model for cultivar classification and identification with reference to oats (*Avena*). II. A probabilistic definition of cultivar groupings and their Bayesian identification. *Canadian Journal of Botany*, **50**, 131–138.

Bianchi A T J, 1931: Een Nieuwe Determinatie-Methode (in Dutch with English summary). *Tectona*, **24**, 884–893.

BIOSIS, 1985: *Zoological Record Search Guide*. BIOSIS, Philadelphia and York.

Bisby F A, 1984: Information services in taxonomy. In *Databases in Systematics*, Allkin R and Bisby F A, (eds) 17–33, Academic Press, London and Orlando.

Bisby F A and Nicholls K W, 1977: Effects of varying character definitions on classification of Genisteae (Leguminosae). *Botanical Journal of the Linnean Society*, **74**, 97–121.

Bonnier G, 1917: *Les Noms des Fleurs par la Méthode Simple*. Librairie Generale, Paris.

Boughey A S, Bridges K W and Ikeda A G, 1968: *An Automated Biological Identification Key*. Research series No.2. Museum of Systematic Biology, University of California, Irvine.

B-P-H see Lawrence *et al.*

Brodman K, Van Woerkom A J, Erdmann A J and Goldstein L S, 1959: Interpretations of symptoms with a data-processing machine. *Archives of Internal Medicine*, **103**, 116–122.

Brohmer P, Ehrmann P and Ulmer G, 1960: *Tierwelt Mitteleuropas*. Quelle and Meyer, Leipzig.

Brough D R and Alexander I F, 1986: The Fossil expert system. *Expert Systems*, **3**, 76–83.

Brown P J, 1977: Functions for selecting tests in diagnostic key construction. *Biometrika*, **64**, 589–596.

Brues C T, Melander A L and Carpenter F M, 1954: *Classification of Insects*. Harvard University Press, Cambridge, Massachusetts.

Burnham W D and Hall A R, 1985: *PROLOG Programming and Applications*. Macmillan, London.

Cadbury DA, Hawkes JG and Readett RC, 1971: *A Computer-mapped Flora*. Academic Press, London and New York.

Cairns Jr. J, Almeida S P and Fujii H, 1982: Automated identification of diatoms. *Bioscience*, **32**, 98–102.

Camin J H and Sokal R R, 1965: A method for deducing branching sequences in phylogeny. *Evolution*, **19**, 311–326.

Campbell I, 1973: Computer identification of the genus *Saccharomyces*. *Journal of General Microbiology*, **77**, 127–135.

Charlwood B V, Morris G S and Grenham M J, 1984: A chemical database for the Leguminosae. In *Databases in Systematics*, Allkin R and Bisby F A, (eds) 201–208, Academic Press, London and Orlando.

Chinery M, 1973: *A Field Guide to the Insects of Britain and Northern Europe*. Collins, London.

Chvatal V, 1979: A greedy heuristic for the set-covering problem. *Mathematics of Operation Research*, **4**, 233–235.

Clapham A R, Tutin T G and Warburg E F, 1962: *Flora of the British Isles*. (2E). Cambridge University Press, Cambridge and London.

Clarke S H, 1937: *The Construction of Keys to the Identification of Timber.*. Progress Report No.4. Forest Products Research Laboratory, HMSO, London.

Claus E P, 1956: *Gathercoal and Wirth's Pharmacognosy*. (3E). Henry Kimpton, London.

Codd E F, 1983: A relational model of data for large shared data banks. *Communications of the A.C.M.*, **26**, 64–69.

Cole A J and Wishart D, 1970: An improved algorithm for the Jardine-Sibson method of generating overlapping clusters. *Computer Journal*, **13**, 156–163.

Correl L, 1977: The application of maximal predictive classification in the Epacridaceae. *Taxon*, **26**, 65–67.

COSMOS Incorporated, 1987: *Advanced Revelation*. Bellevue, Washington and New York.

Cotton G, 1973: *The Rugose Coral Genera*. Elsevier, Amsterdam.

Cowan S T and Steel K J, 1960: A device for the identification of micro-organisms. *Lancet*, **1**, 1172–1173.

—— 1965: *Manual for the Identification of Medical Bacteria*. Cambridge University Press, Cambridge and London.

Crawford R M M and Wishart D, 1967: A rapid multivariate method for the detection and classification of groups of ecologically related species. *Journal of Ecology*, **55**, 505–524.

Creighton R A and Crockett J J, 1971: SELGEM; a system for collection management. *Information Systems Innovations*, **(3)**, 1–24. Smithsonian Institution, Washington DC.

Croft D J, 1972: Is computerised diagnosis possible? *Computers and Biomedical Research*, **5**, 351–367.

Cronquist A, 1987: A botanical critique of cladism. *Botanical Review*, **53**, 1–52.

Crosby M R and Magill R E, 1989: *TROPICOS, a botanical database system at the Missouri Botanical Garden*. Missouri Botanical Garden.

Dallwitz M J, 1974: A flexible computer program for generating diagnostic keys. *Systematic Zoology*, **23**, 50–57.

—— 1980: *User's Guide to the DELTA System: a general system for encoding taxonomic descriptions*. Available from the author free of charge. CSIRO Division of Entomology, Canberra, Australia.

—— 1984: Automatic typesetting of computer-generated keys and descriptions. In *Databases in Systematics*, Allkin R and Bisby F A, (eds) 279–290, Academic Press, London and Orlando.

Date C J, 1981: *An Introduction to Database Systems*. Addison-Wesley, Wokingham and Reading (Massachusetts).

—— 1987: *A Guide to the SQL Standard*. Addison-Wesley, Wokingham and Reading (Massachusetts).

Davies R G, 1981: Information theory and character selection in the numerical taxonomy of some male Diaspididae (Hemiptera: Coccoidea). *Systematic Entomology*, **6**, 149–178.

Davis P H and Cullen J, 1965: *The Identification of Flowering Plant Families*. Oliver and Boyd, Edinburgh and London.

Davis P H and Heywood V H, 1963: *Principles of Angiosperm Taxonomy*. Oliver and Boyd, Edinburgh and London.

Del Amo S, 1979: *Plantas medicinales del estado de Verucruz*. INIREB, Jalapa, Veracruz, Mexico.

Derrick L N, Jermy A C and Paul A M, 1987: Checklist of European pteridophytes. *Sommerfeltia*, **6**, i–xx, 1–94.

Duke J A, 1969: On tropical tree seedlings I. Seeds, seedlings, systems and systematics. *Annals of the Missouri Botanical Garden*, **56(2)**, 125–161.

Duncan T and Meacham C A, 1986: MEKA Version 1.1. A general purpose multiple-entry key algorithm. Herbarium, University of California, Berkeley.

Dunn G and Everitt B S, 1982: *An Introduction to Mathematical Taxonomy*. Cambridge University Press, Cambridge and London.

Dussart G B J, 1980: A key to statistical methods for biologists. *School Science Review*, **66**, 476–489.

Ellis B F and Messina A, 1940 (et seq.): *Catalogue of Foraminifera*. American Natural History Museum, New York.

Essex B J, 1975: *Diagnostic Pathways in Clinical Medicine*. Churchill Livingstone, Edinburgh.

Estabrook G F, 1967: An information theory model for character analysis. *Taxon*, **16**, 86–96.

—— 1968: A general solution in partial orders to the Camin-Sokal model in phylogeny. *Journal of Theoretical Biology*, **21**, 421–438.

Esterre P, Vignes R and Lebbe J, 1987: Identification assisstée par ordinateur: application aux levures pathogènes. *Bulletin de la Société Française de Mycologie Médicale*, **16**, 117–120.

Evans D F, Hill M O and Ward S D, 1977: *A dichotomous key to British Submontane Vegetation*. Occasional Paper No.1, Institute of Terrestrial Ecology, Bangor.

Evans W H, 1949: *A Catalogue of the Hesperidae*. British Museum (Natural History), London.

F.A.O., 1973: *Species identification Sheets for Fishery Purposes*. F.A.O., Rome.

Farr E R, Leussink J A and Stafleu F A, (eds), 1979: *Index Nominum Genericorum (Plantarum)*. Bohn, Scheltema and Holkema, Utrecht and Dr. Junk, The Hague.

Farris J S, 1970: Methods for computing Wagner Trees. *Systematic Zoology*, **19**, 83–92.

—— 1979: The information content of the phylogenetic system. *Systematic Zoology*. **28**, 483–519.

—— 1988: HENNIG 86 reference. Department of Ecology and Evolution, State University of New York, Stony Brook.

Feigenbaum E A, 1979: Themes and case studies of knowledge engineering. In *Expert Systems in the Micro-electronic age*, Michie D, (ed.) 3–25, Edinburgh University Press, Edinburgh.

Feinstein A, 1958: *Foundations of Information Theory*. McGraw Hill, New York.

Felsenstein J, 1978a: The number of evolutionary trees. *Systematic Zoology*, **27**, 27–33.

—— 1978b: Cases in which parsimony or compatibility methods will be positively misleading. *Systematic Zoology*, **27**, 401–410.

—— 1979: Alternative methods of phylogenetic inference and their interrelationship. *Systematic Zoology*, **28**, 49–62.

—— 1984: The statistical approach to inferring evolutionary trees and what it tells us about parsimony and compatibility. In *Cladistics: perspectives on the reconstruction of evolutionary history*, Duncan T and Stuessy T F, (eds) 169–191, Columbia University Press, New York.

—— 1985a: Confidence limits on phylogenies: an approach using the bootstrap. *Evolution*, **39**, 783–791.

—— 1985b: *PHYLIP, phylogeny inference package*. Department of Genetics SK-50, Washington University, Seattle.

Fiala K L, 1984: *CLINCH, program for cladistic inference by compatibility*. Department of Ecology and Evolution, State University of New York, Stony Brook.

Fink W L, 1986: Microcomputers and phylogenetic analysis. *Science*, **234**, 1135–1139.

Fitter A H, 1980: Hybridisation in Epilobium (Onagraceae): the effect of clearance and the re-establishment of fen carr. *Biological Journal of the Linnean Society*, **13**, 331–339.

Flesness N R, Garnatz P G and Seal U S, 1984: ISIS – an international specimen information system. In *Databases in Systematics*, Allkin R and Bisby F A, (eds) 103–112, Academic Press, London and Orlando.

Forget P M, Lebbe J, Puig H, Vignes R and Hideux M, 1986: Microcomputer-aided identification: an application to trees from French Guiana. *Botanical Journal of the Linnean Society*, **93**, 205–223.

Fortuner R, 1986: A better assessment of variability of qualitative characters for the computer identification program NEMAID. *Revue Nématol.*, **9**, 277–279.

Fortuner R and Wong Y, 1984: Review of the genus *Helicotylenchus* Steiner, 1945. I: A computer program for identification of the species. *Revue Nématol.*, **7**, 385–392.

Freemon F R, 1972: Medical diagnosis, comparison of human and computer logic. *Biomedical Computing*, **3**, 217–221.

Gaspard D and Mullon C, 1980: Etude de la différenciation sur trois populations de térébratules biplissées du Cénomanien. *Cahiers de l'Analyse des Données*, **5**, 193–211.

Gauld I D, 1980: An analysis of classification. Ophion genus group. *Systematic Entomology*, **5**, 59–82.

Geesink R, Leeuwenberg A J M, Ridsdale C E and Veldkamp J F, 1981: *Thonner's analytical key to the families of flowering plants*. Leiden Botanical Series, **5**. PUDOC, Centre for Agricultural Publishing and Documentation, Wageningen, and Leiden University Press, The Hague.

Germeraad J H and Muller J, 1972: *Computer-based Numerical Coding System for the Description of Pollen Grains and Spores*. National Museum of Geology and Mineralogy, Leiden.

Gilmour J S L, 1937: A taxonomic problem. *Nature*, **139**, 1040–1042.

Gómez-Pompa A, Moreno N P, Gama L, Sosa V and Allkin R, 1984: Flora of Veracruz: progress and prospects. In *Databases in Systematics*, Allkin R and Bisby F A, (eds) 165–174, Academic Press, London and Orlando.

Gómez-Pompa A and Nevling Jr. L I, 1973: The use of electronic data processing methods in the flora of Veracruz program. *Contributions of the Gray Herbarium*, **203**, 49–64.

Goodall A, 1985: *The Guide to Expert Systems*. Learned Information, Oxford and New Jersey.

Goodman D, 1987: *The complete HyperCard handbook*. Bantam Books, Toronto, New York, London, Sydney and Auckland.

Gordon A D, 1981: *Classification: methods for the exploratory analysis of multivariate data*. Chapman and Hall, London and New York.

Gordon J and Shortliffe E H, 1985: A method for managing evidential reasoning in a hierarchical hypothesis space. *Artificial Intelligence*, **26**, 323–357.

Gower J C, 1966: Some distance properties of latent root and vector methods used in multivariate analysis. *Biometrika*, **53**, 325–338.

—— 1971: A general coefficient of similarity and some of its properties. *Biometrics*, **27**, 857–871.

—— 1973: Classification problems. *Proceedings of International Statistics Institute, 39th session (Vienna)* 471–477.

—— 1974: Maximal predictive classification. *Biometrics*, **30**, 643–654.

Gower J C and Payne R W, 1975: A comparison of different criteria for selecting binary tests in diagnostic keys. *Biometrika*, **62**, 665–672.

Graham R L and Foulds L R, 1982: Unlikelihood that minimal phylogenies for a realistic biological study can be constructed in reasonable computational time. *Mathematical Biosciences*, **60**, 133–142.

Greenacre M J, 1984: *Theory and Applications of Correspondence Analysis*. Academic Press, London and Orlando.

Grew N, 1682: Appendix to Part 2 of Book 4 of *The Anatomy of Plants with an idea of a Philosophical History of Plants*. W. Rawlins (printer).

Guittoneau G G and Roux M, 1977: Sur la taxinomie du genre Erodium. *Cahiers de l'Analyse des Données*, **2**, 97–113.

Gyllenberg H G, 1963: A general method for deriving determination schemes for random collections of microbial isolates. *Annals of the Finnish Academy of Sciences, ser. A, IV. Biology*, **69**, 1–23.

Gyllenberg H G and Niemelä T K, 1975: New approaches to microbial identification. In *Biological Identification with Computers*, Pankhurst R J, (ed.) 121–136, Academic Press, London and Orlando.

Hall A V, 1973: The use of a computer-based system of aids for classification. *Contributions of the Bolus Herbarium*, **6**, University of Cape Town.

Hall N and Johnston R D, 1954: *Card sorting key for the identification of eucalypts*. Forestry and Timber Bureau, Canberra.

Hansen B and Rahn K, 1969: Determination of angiosperm families by means of a punched card system. *Dansk Botanisk Arkiv*, **26**.

Harris T M, 1961: *Yorkshire Jurassic Flora*. British Museum (Natural History), London.

Hayes-Roth F, Waterman D and Lenat D, (eds) 1983: *Building Expert Systems*. Addison-Wesley, Wokingham and Reading (Massachusetts).

Hedge I C and Lamond J C, 1972: Multi-access key to the Turkish genera (of Umbelliferae). In *Flora of Turkey*, Davis P H, (ed.) 280–288, Edinburgh University Press, Edinburgh.

Hendy M D and Penny D, 1982: Branch and bound algorithms to determine minimal evolutionary trees. *Mathematical Biosciences*, **59**, 277–290.

Hennig W, 1965: Phylogenetic systematics. *Annual Review of Entomology*, **10**, 97–116.

—— 1966: *Phylogenetic Systematics*. University of Illinois Press, Urbana.

Heywood V H, Moore D M, Derrick L N, Mitchell K A and Van Scheepen J, 1984: The European taxonomic, floristic and biosystematic documentation system – an introduction. In *Databases in Systematics*, Allkin R and Bisby F A, (eds), Academic Press, London and Orlando.

Hill C R and Camus J M, 1986: Evolutionary cladistics of marattialean ferns. *Bulletin of the British Museum (Natural History), Botany Series*, **14**, 219–300.

Hill M O, Bunce R G H and Shaw M W, 1975: Indicator species analysis, a divisive polythetic method of classification, and its application to a survey of native pinewoods in Scotland. *Journal of Ecology* **63**, 597–613.

ILDIS, 1988–: *Newsletter*. ILDIS Coordinating Centre, Biology Department, University of Southampton.

Index, Herbariorum *see* Stafleu, 1981.

Index Kewensis, 1893–: Clarendon Press, Oxford.

ING, Index Nominum Genericorum, *see* Farr *et al*, 1979.

Jardine N and Sibson R, 1968: The construction of hierarchic and non-hierarchic classifications. *Computer Journal*, **11**, 177–184.

—— 1971: *Mathematical Taxonomy*. Wiley, London.

Jeffrey C, 1989: *Biological Nomenclature*. (3E). Edward Arnold, London.

Jolliffe G N and Jolliffe G O, 1976: Computer-aided identification of powdered vegetable drugs. *Analyst*, **101**, 622–633.

Kautz W H, 1968: Fault testing and diagnosis in combinatorial digital circuits. *IEEE Transactions in Computing*, **17**, 352–366.

Kernigan B W and Ritchie D M, 1978: *The C Programming Language*. Prentice Hall, New Jersey.

Kerrich G J, Hawksworth D L and Sims R W, 1978: *Key works to the Fauna and Flora of the British Isles and Northwestern Europe*. For the Systematics Association by Academic Press, London and Orlando.

Kew Record, 1971–: *The Kew Record of Taxonomic Literature*. HMSO, Royal Botanic Gardens, Kew.

Kluge A G and Farris J S, 1969: Quantitative phyletics and the evolution of anurans. *Systematic Zoology*, **18**, 1–32.

Kožuharov S, 1976: *Jurinea*. In *Flora Europea*, Tutin T G *et al*, (eds) **4**, 218–220, Cambridge University Press, Cambridge and London.

Krombein K V, Mello J F and Crockett J J, 1974: The North American Hymenoptera catalog: a pioneering effort in computerized publication. *Bulletin of the Entomological Society of America*, **20**, 24–29.

Kruskal J B, 1964a: Multidimensional scaling by optimizing goodness of fit to a non-metric hypothesis. *Psychometrika*, **29**, 2–17.
—— 1964b: Nonmetric multidimensional scaling: a numerical method. *Psychometrika*, **29**, 28–42.
Kudo R R, 1966: *Protozoology*. (5E). C.C. Thomas, Springfield, Illinois.
Lamark J B P, 1778: *Flore Française*. (1E). Imprimerie Royal, Paris.
Lance G N and Williams W T, 1967: A general theory of classificatory sorting strategies. I Hierarchical systems. *Computer Journal*, **9**, 373–380.
—— 1968: Note on a new information-statistic classificatory program. *Computer Journal*, **11**, 195.
Lapasha C A and Wheeler E A, 1987: A microcomputer based system for computer-aided wood identification. *IAWA Bulletin, new series*, **8**, 347–354.
Lawrence G H M, 1951: *Taxonomy of Vascular Plants*. Macmillan, New York.
Lawrence G H M, Buchheim A F G, Daniels G S and Dolezal H, (eds), 1968: *Botanico Periodicum Huntianum*. Hunt Botanical Library, Pittsburgh, Pennsylvania.
Lebbe J, 1984: *Manuel d'utilisation du logiciel XPER*. Micro Application, Paris.
—— 1986: Les champignons identifiés par ordinateur. *Science et Vie*, Oct. 1986, 126–130.
Lebbe J, Vignes R and Dedet J P, 1987: *Identification assistée par ordinateur des phlébotomes de la Guyane Française*. Institut Pasteur de la Guyane Française.
Leenhouts P W, 1968: A guide to the practice of herbarium taxonomy. *Regnum Vegetabile*, **58**.
Lefkovitch L P, 1985: Entropy and set covering. *Information Sciences*, **36**, 283–294.
Le Quesne W J, 1974: The uniquely evolved character concept and its cladistic application. *Systematic Zoology*, **23**, 513–517.
Lewis H R and Papadimitriou C H, 1978: The efficiency of algorithms. *Scientific American*, **238(1)**, 96–109.
Linnaeus C, 1736: *Clavis Classium in Systemate Phytologorum*. In *Bibliotheca Botanica*, Amsterdam.
Lobanov A J, Schilow W F and Nikritin L M, 1981: Zur Anwendung von Computern für die Determination in der Entomologie. *Deutsche Entomologie Zeitung*, **28**, 29–43.
Lucas G, 1989: Index Kewensis on computer. *Taxon*, **38**, 529–530.
Mackinder D C, 1984: The database of the IUCN conservation monitoring centre. In *Databases in Systematics*, Allkin R and Bisby F A, (eds) 91–102, Academic Press, London and Orlando.
Maddison W and Maddison D, 1987: *MacClade for the Apple Macintosh*. Museum of Comparative Zoology, Harvard University, Cambridge, Massachusettes.
Mamdani E H and Efstathiou H J, 1985: Higher-order logics for handling uncertainty in expert systems. *International Journal of Man-Machine Studies*, **22**, 283–293.
Mascherpa J M and Bocquet G, 1981: Deux programmes interactif de détermination automatique. Une idée, un but. *Candollea*, **36**, 463–483.
Mayr E, 1969: *Principles of Systematic Zoology*. McGraw-Hill, New York.
Meacham C A, 1980: Phylogeny of the Berberidaceae with an evaluation of classifications. *Systematic Botany*, **5**, 149–172.
—— 1984: Evaluating characters by character compatibility analysis. In *Cladistics: perspectives on the reconstruction of evolutionary history*, Duncan T and Stuessy T F, (eds) 152–165, Columbia University Press, New York.
Meikle R D, 1971: The history of the Index Kewensis. *Biological Journal of the Linnean Society*, **3**, 295–299.
—— 1980: *Draft Index of Author Abbreviations*. HMSO, Royal Botanic Gardens, Kew.
Mendel J M and Fu K S, (eds), 1970: *Adaptive Learning and Pattern Recognition*. Academic Press, London and Orlando.
Metcalfe C R and Chalk L, 1950: *Anatomy of the Dicotyledons*. Clarendon Press, Oxford.
Michalski R S and Chilausky R L, 1980: Knowledge acquisition by encoding expert rules versus computer induction from examples: a case study involving soybean pathology. *International Journal of Man-machine Studies*, **12**, 63–87.
Mickevich M F, 1978: Taxonomic congruence. *Systematic Zoology*, **27** 143–158.
Microsoft Corporation, 1985: *Microsoft Paintbrush User's Guide*. Microsoft, Redmond, Washington.

Minsky M and Papert S, 1969: *Perceptrons*. Chapters 10 and 11. MIT Press, Cambridge, Massachusetts.

Morin N R, Whetstone R D, Wilken D and Tomlinson K L, (eds), 1989: *Floristics for the 21st century*. Proceedings of May 1988 Workshop (Alexandria, Virginia), Missouri Botanical Garden, St. Louis.

Morison R, 1672: *Plantarum Umbelliferarum Distributio Nova*. Oxford, Sheldonian Theatre.

Morris J W, 1974: Progress in the computerisation of herbarium procedures. *Bothalia*, **11**, 349–354.

Morse L E, 1974: Computer programs for specimen identification, key construction and description printing. *Publications of the Museum of Michigan State University, Biology*, **5**.

—— 1975: Recent advances in the theory and practice of biological specimen identification. In *Biological Identification with Computers*, Pankhurst R J, (ed.) 11–52, Academic Press, London and Orlando.

Morse L E, Pankhurst R J and Rypka E W, 1975: A glossary of computer-assisted biological specimen identification. In *Biological Identification with Computers*, Pankhurst R J, (ed.), 315–330, Academic Press, London and Orlando.

Nash F A, 1960: Diagnostic reasoning and the logoscope. *Lancet*, **1**, 1442–1446.

Nelson P F, 1972: *Analytical Microscopy of Vegetable Materials*. Available from the author.

Newell I M, 1970: Construction and use of tabular keys. *Pacific Insects*, **12**, 25–37.

Nimis P L, Feoli E and Pignatti S, 1984: The network of databanks for the Italian flora and vegetation. In *Databases in Systematics*, Allkin R and Bisby F A, (eds) 113–124, Academic Press, London and Orlando.

Nooteboom HP, 1975: *Revision of the Symplocaceae of the Old World*. PhD Thesis, Leiden.

Ogden E C, 1943: The broad-leaved species of *Potamogeton* of North America north of Mexico. *Rhodora*, **45**, 57–105.

Olds R J, 1970: Identification of bacteria with the aid of an improved information sorter. In *Automation, Mechanisation and Data Handling in Microbiology*, Baillie A and Gilbert A J, (eds) 85–89, Academic Press, London and Orlando.

Oracle Corporation, 1987: *SQL*Plus user's guide*. Oracle Corporation, Belmont, California.

Osborne D V, 1963: Some aspects of the theory of dichotomous keys. *New Phytologist*, **62**, 144–160.

Page R D M, 1988: Quantitative cladistic biogeography, constructing and comparing area cladograms. *Systematic Zoology*, **37**, 254–270.

Pankhurst R J, 1970: A computer program for generating diagnostic keys. *Computer Journal*, **12**, 145–151.

—— 1971: Botanical keys generated by computer. *Watsonia*, **8**, 357–368.

—— 1975: Identification by matching. In *Biological Identification with Computers*, Pankhurst R J, (ed.) 79–91, Academic Press, London and Orlando.

—— 1978a: *Biological Identification. The principles and practice of identification methods in biology*. Edward Arnold, London.

—— 1978b: The printing of taxonomic descriptions by computer. *Taxon*, **27**, 65–68.

—— 1983a: An improved algorithm for finding diagnostic taxonomic descriptions. *Mathematical Biosciences*, **65**, 209–218.

—— 1983b: The construction of a floristic database. *Taxon*, **32**, 193–202.

—— 1984: A review of herbarium catalogues. In *Databases in Systematics*, Allkin R and Bisby F A, (eds) 155–164, Academic Press, London and Orlando.

—— 1988a: Database design for monographs and floras. *Taxon*, **37**, 733–746.

—— 1988b: An interactive program for the construction of identification keys. *Taxon*, **37**, 747–755.

—— 1989: A computer program with colour graphics to identify orchids. *Orchid Review*, **97**, 53–55, 67.

Pankhurst R J and Aitchison R R, 1975a: A computer program to construct polyclaves. In *Biological Identification with Computers*, Pankhurst R J, (ed.) 73–78, Academic Press, London and Orlando.

—— 1975b: An on-line identification program. In *Biological Identification with Computers*, Pankhurst R J, (ed.) 181–194, Academic Press, London and Orlando.

Pankhurst R J and Allinson J M, 1985: *British Grasses, a punched card key to grasses in the vegetative state*. Field Studies Council Occasional Publication No.10, and British Museum (Natural History), London.

Pankhurst R J and Chater A O, 1988 : Sedges of the British Isles. *BSBI Computer Key No.1*, version 2 (illustrated). Botanical Society of the British Isles, Natural History Museum, London.

Payne R W, 1975: Genkey: a program for constructing diagnostic keys. In *Biological Identification with Computers*, Pankhurst R J, (ed.) 65–72, Academic Press, London and Orlando.

—— 1980: Alternative characters in identification keys. *Classification Society Bulletin*, **4**, 16–21.

—— 1981: Selection criteria for the construction of efficient diagnostic keys. *Journal of Statistical Planning and Inference*, **5**, 27–36.

—— 1984: Computer construction and typesetting of identification keys. *New Phytologist*, **96**, 631–634.

Payne R W and Dixon T J, 1984: A study of selection criteria for constructing identification keys. *COMPSTAT Proceedings in computational statistics*, Physica Verlag, Vienna, 148–153.

Payne R W, Lamacraft R R and White R P, 1981: The dual polyclave: an aid to more efficient identification. *New Phytologist*, **87**, 121–126.

Payne R W and Preece D A, 1977: Incorporating checks against observer error into identification keys. *New Phytologist*, **79**, 201–207.

—— 1980: Identification keys and diagnostic tables: a review. *Journal of the Royal Statistical Society, series A*, **143**, 253–292.

Pearson R G and Wheeler E A, 1981: Computer identification of hardwood species. *IAWA Bulletin, new series*, **2**, 37–40.

Perring F H and Walters S M, 1962: *Atlas of the British Flora*. Botanical Society of the British Isles and Thomas Nelson, London.

Phillips E W J, 1948: Identification of Softwoods by their Microscopic Structure. *Forest Products Research Bulletin*, **22**, HMSO, London.

Platnick N, 1987: An empirical comparison of microcomputer programs. *Cladistics*, **3**, 121–144.

Podani J, 1988: SYN-TAX III user's manual. *Abstracts Botanica*, **12**, Supplement I.

Quinlan J R, 1979: Discovering rules by induction from large collections of examples. In *Expert Systems in the Microelectronic age*, Michie D, (ed.) 168–186, Edinburgh University Press, Edinburgh.

—— 1985: *Decision trees and multi-valued attributes*. Technical Report 85.4, University of Technology, Sydney.

Radford A E, Dickinson W C, Massey J R and Bell C R, 1974: *Vascular Plant Systematics*. Harper and Row, New York.

Rao C K and Pankhurst R J, 1986: *A polyclave to the Monocotyledonous Families of the World. A computer generated identification key*. British Museum (Natural History), London.

Ray J, 1686: *Historia Piscium*. Oxford, Sheldonian Theatre.

Rhoades F, 1986: *PC-TAXON: a taxonomic database, user's guide*. COMPress, Wentworth, New Hampshire.

RHODNIUS Incorporated, 1986: *Empress database systems, product overview*. Rhodnius Inc., Toronto.

Ritchie, J, Brodlie P and Harden R M, 1975: Drug identification using punched feature cards. *Lancet*, March 8th, 552–555.

Rohlf F J, 1982: Consensus indices for comparing classifications. *Mathematical-Biosciences*, **59**, 1341–44.

—— 1988: *NTSYS – Numerical Taxonomy and Multivariate Analysis System*, (version 1.50). Applied Biostatistics Incorporated, Setauket, New York.

Romesburg H C, 1984: *Cluster Analysis for Researchers*. Lifetime Learning Publications, Belmont, California.

Ross G J S, 1975: Rapid techniques for automatic identification. In *Biological Identification with Computers*, Pankhurst R J, (ed.) 93–102, Academic Press, London and Orlando.

Russell G E G and Arnold T H, 1989: Fifteen years with the computer: assessment of the PRECIS taxonomic system. *Taxon*, **38**, 178–195.

Russell G E G and Gonsalves P, 1984: PRECIS – a curatorial and biogeographic system. In *Databases in Systematics*, Allkin R and Bisby F A, (eds) 137–153, Academic Press, London and Orlando.

Rypka E W, 1971: Truth table classification and identification. *Space Life Sciences*, **3**, 135–156.

—— 1975: Pattern recognition and microbial identification, In *Biological Identification with Computers*, Pankhurst R J, (ed.) 153–180, Academic Press, London and Orlando.

Rypka E W, Clapper W E, Bowen I G and Babb R, 1967: A model for the identification of bacteria. *Journal of General Microbiology*, **46**, 407–424.

Shafer G, 1976: *A Mathematical Theory of Evidence*. Princeton University Press, New Jersey.

Shortliffe E H, 1976: *Computer-based Medical Consultations: MYCIN*. Elsevier, Amsterdam.

Shultz L M, 1975: Program CDKEY. In *Biological Identification with Computers*, Pankhurst R J, (ed.) 306, Academic Press, London and Orlando.

Sieg J, 1984: Fact documentation and literature database for the Crustacean order Tanaidacea. In *Databases in Systematics*, Allkin R and Bisby F A, (eds) 125–136, Academic Press, London and Orlando.

Sinker C D, 1975: A lateral key to common grasses. *Bulletin of the Shropshire Wildlife Trust*, **31**, 11–18.

Sinnott Q P, 1982: Polyclave keying with one card per character. *Taxon*, **31**, 277–279.

Skov F, 1989a: *HyperTaxonomy – a new tool for revisional work and a revision of Geonoma (Palmae) in Ecuador*. Ph.D. thesis, University of Aarhus, Denmark.

—— 1989b: HyperTaxonomy – a new computer tool for revisional work. *Taxon*, **38**, 582–590.

Smith D G W and Leibovitz D P, 1986: *MiniDent User's Manual*. Computer Services, University of Alberta, Canada.

Sneath P H A, 1975: Cladistic representation of reticulate evolution. *Sytematic Zoology*, **24**, 360–368.

—— 1979: BASIC program for identification of an unknown with presence-absence data against an identification matrix of percent positive characters. *Computing and Geosciences*, **5**, 195–213.

Sneath P H A and Hansell R I C, 1985: Naturalness and predictivity of classifications. *Biological Journal of the Linnean Society*, **24,,** 217–231.

Sneath P H A and Sokal R R, 1973: *Numerical Taxonomy*. Freeman and Co., San Francisco.

Sokal R R and Rohlf F J, 1962: Cophenetic comparisons of dendrograms. *Taxon*, **11**, 33–40.

Sporne K R, 1954: Statistics and the evolution of dicotyledons. *Evolution*, **8**, 55–64.

Stace C A, 1975: *Hybridisation and the Flora of the British Isles*. Academic Press, London and Orlando.

—— 1987: Hybridisation and the plant species. In *Differentiation Patterns in Higher Plants*, Urbanska K M, (ed.) 115–127, Academic Press, London and Orlando.

—— 1989: *Plant Taxonomy and Biosystematics*. (2E). Edward Arnold, London.

Stafleu F A, (ed.), 1981: *Index Herbariorum*. (7E). Bohn, Scheltema and Holkema, Utrecht/Antwerpen and Dr W Junk, The Hague/Boston.

Stafleu F A and Cowan R S. 1976–1988: *Taxonomic Literature*. (2E). Bohn, Scheltema and Holkema, Utrecht/Antwerpen and Dr W Junk, The Hague/Boston.

Stone, N D, Coulson R N, Frisbie R E and Loh D K, 1986: Expert systems in entomology: three approaches to problem-solving. *Bulletin of the Entomological Society of America*, **32**, 161–166.

Stuessy T F and Crisci J V, 1984: Problems in the determination of evolutionary directionality of character-state change for phylogenetic reconstruction. In *Cladistics: perspectives on the reconstruction of evolutionary history*, Duncan T and Stuessy T F, (eds), 71–87, Columbia University Press, New York.

Swofford D L, 1983: *PAUP, phylogenetic analysis using parsimony*. Illinois Natural History Survey, Illinois.

Sylvester-Bradley P C and Siveter D J, (eds), 1973: *A Stereo-Atlas of Ostracod Shells*. Department of Geology, University of Leicester.

Takhtajan A L, 1980: Outline of the classification of flowering plants (Magnoliophyta). *Botanical Review*, **46**, 225–359.

Taylor M, 1985: *PICK for users*. Blackwell Scientific Publications, Oxford.

Thompson B A and Thompson W A, 1985: Inside an expert System. *Byte*, April 1985, 315–330.

Thonnat M and Gandelin M H, 1988: An expert system for the automatic classification and description of zooplankton from monocular images. *9th International Conference on Pattern Recognition (Rome)*.

Tutin T G, 1980: *Umbellifers of the British Isles*. Botanical Society of the British Isles, Handbook No. 2, London.

Tutin T G, Heywood V H, Burges N A, Valentine D H, Walters S M and Webb D A (Eds), 1964–1988: *Flora Europaea*, Cambridge University Press.

Von Hayek C M F, 1990: A reclassification of the *Melanotus* group of genera (Coleoptera: Elateridae). *Bulletin of the Natural History Museum, Entomology*, **59**, 37–115.

Voss E G, 1952: The history of keys and phylogenetic trees in systematic biology. *Journal of the Scientific Laboratories, Denison University*, **43(1)**, 1–25.

Wagner Jr. J H, 1963: Biosystematics and taxonomic categories in lower vascular plants. *Regnum Vegetabile*, **27**, 63–71.

Walker D, Milne P, Gubby J and Williams J, 1968: The computer assisted storage and retrieval of pollen morphological data. *Pollen et Spores*, **10**, 251–262.

Walters S M, 1975: Traditional methods of biological identification. In *Biological Identification with Computers*, Pankhurst R J, (ed.) 3–8, Academic Press, London and Orlando.

Ward J H, 1963: Hierarchical grouping to optimize an objective function. *Journal of the American Statistical Association*, **58**, 236–244.

Watson L and Dallwitz M J, 1988: *Grass genera of the world*. Research School of Biological Sciences, Australian National University, Canberra.

Watson L and Milne P, 1972: A flexible system for automatic generation of special purpose dichotomous keys, and its application to Australian grass genera. *Australian Journal of Botany*, **20**, 331–352.

Weber W A and Nelson P P, 1972: *Random-access Key to Genera of Colorado Mosses*. University of Colorado Museum, Boulder.

Whalley P E S, 1976: *Tropical Leaf Moths*. British Museum (Natural History), London.

Wiley E O, 1981: *The Theory and Practice of Phylogenetic Systematics*. Wiley, New York.

Wilkins J, 1668: *An essay towards a real character and a philosophical language*. Royal Society, London.

Willcox W R and Lapage S P, 1972: Automatic construction of diagnostic tables. *Computer Journal*, **15(3)**, 263–267.

Willcox W R, Lapage S P, Bascomb S and Curtis M A, 1973: Identification of bacteria by computer: theory and programming. *Journal of General Microbiology*, **77**, 317–330.

Willcox W R, Lapage S P and Holmes B, 1980: A review of numerical methods in bacterial identification. *Antonie van Leeuwenhoek*, **46**, 233–299.

Williams W T and Lambert J M, 1959: Multivariate methods in plant ecology. I. Association analysis in plant communities. *Journal of Ecology*, **47**, 83–101.

Wilson J B and Partridge T R, 1986: Interactive plant identification. *Taxon*, **35**, 1–12.

Winfield P J and Green F N, 1984: The use of a descriptive database as an aid to assessing the distinctness of pea cultivars (*Pisum sativum* L.). In *Databases in Systematics*, Allkin R and Bisby F A, (eds) 189–200, Academic Press, London and Orlando.

Wishart D, 1987: *CLUSTAN User Manual*. (4E). Computing Laboratory, University of St. Andrews, Scotland.

Useful addresses

Applied Biostatistics Inc.
3 Heritage Lane
Setauket
New York 11733
USA

BIOSIS
2100 Arch Street
Philadelphia
Pennysylvania 19103–1399
USA

and

Garforth House
54 Micklegate
York
YO1 1LF
England

M J Dallwitz
CSIRO Division of Entomology
P O Box 1700
Canberra
ACT 2601
Australia

Harvard University
Museum of Comparative Zoology
Cambridge
Massachusetts 02138
USA

ILDIS Coordinating Centre
Biology Department
The University
Southampton
SO9 3TU
England

Illinois Natural History Survey
607 East Peabody Drive
Champaign
Illinois 61820
USA

P F Nelson
114 Corsebar Drive
Paisley
Scotland

RHODNIUS Inc.
250 Bloor Street East
Toronto
Canada

TDWG
(Taxonomic Databases Working Group)
Missouri Botanical Garden
P O Box 299
St. Louis
MO 63166
USA

State University of New York
Department of Ecology and Evolution
Stony Brook
New York 11790
USA

University of Idaho
Moscow
Idaho 83843
USA

University of Washington
Department of Genetics
Seattle
Washington 98195
USA

University of Technology
Sydney
NSW 2007
Australia

Appendix

Estimates of the usefulness of characters

This section describes two measures of the usefulness of characters which are widely used in taxonomy. Questions of the convenience, cost or reliability of using the characters are ignored; only their ability to separate taxa from one another is considered here.

One such measure is the *separation number*, or the *separation coefficient*. As originally proposed by Gyllenberg (1963) for a character with two states, the separation $S = n_1 n_2$, where n_1 is the number of taxa showing state 1 and n_2 is the number of taxa showing state 2. If none of the taxa is variable, then $n_1 + n_2 = N$, the number of taxa. Hence the equation

$$S = n_1 (N - n_1)$$

is a function of n_1 (or n_2) only, and is greatest when $n_1 = N/2$. This is the situation where the character divides the available taxa into two equal groups, which would be ideal for a character being used to construct a dichotomous key.

This could be generalised to characters with more than two states, but it is then inconvenient to compare binary with multi–state characters because S ranges over different values, and it needs to be normalised by dividing by some number so that S varies only between 0 and 1 for any kind of character.

Another way of looking at this is to define a *separation coefficient*, s. This is obtained by looking at all possible pairs of taxa, to see whether the character separates each pair or not.

$$s = \frac{\text{No. of pairs of taxa separated}}{\text{Total no. of pairs}}$$

This is a property of the character, relative only to a given set of taxa.

For N taxa, the number of possible different pairs is the number of combinations of two out of N, or $^N C_2$, which is $N(N-1)/2$. For a binary character, the maximum value of s is approximately 1/2, for a 3–state character 2/3, and so on, so that for an m–state character, the maximum is roughly $(m-1)/m$. This approximation is close, and is more nearly exact for a large number of taxa. Hence s varies between zero and $(m-1)/m$, which is less than 1. One could make all the values of s lie in the same range by defining s' as $ms/(m-1)$, so that s' lies between 0 and 1 always. However, one could argue that the amount of useful information in a character ought to increase with m, so it may be best to use s and not s'.

The coefficient s can equally well be defined for two or more characters at once. As the pairs of taxa are considered, one can examine whether any one of the relevant characters, or some combination of them distinguishes the two taxa. For two characters a and b, s_{ab} will usually be larger than s_a or s_b alone, unless a and b have exactly the same distribution of states over taxa, or if either s_a or s_b is zero.

Another measure for the usefulness of characters is the *information statistic*. This was originally worked out for problems of errors in the transmission of signals in telecommunication. There is a mathematical derivation of it (e.g. Feinstein 1958) which is remarkable for the amount that can be deduced from very simple assumptions. This is not all explained here but some background is provided.

Suppose we consider a binary character. The proportion p_1 of state 1 for a group of taxa is n_1/N. Likewise, for state 2, $p_2 = n_2/N$, and since $n_1 + n_2 = N$, $p_2 = 1 - p_1$. The 'information' we get from seeing state 1 on a specimen is the effect this fact has on our opinion of what taxon we think we have. If p_1 was 1 (i.e. all taxa show character state 1 only), then on seeing state 1 we would gain no information at all. If $I(p_1)$ stands for the 'information' gained from observing state 1, then the average 'information' H we get by observing this character is:

$$H = p_1 I(p_1) + p_2 I(p_2)$$

Evidently, if we observe the same set of characters but in a different order, the final gain of information ought to be the same regardless of the sequence. Expressed in the above rather general terms, that is about enough to decide what the function H must be, and it is:

$$H = - p_1 \log p_1 - p_2 \log p_2$$

or, for a character with m states;

$$H = - \sum_{i=1}^{m} p_i \log p_i$$

The minus sign is put in because $p_i < 1$, and all values of $\log p_i$ are negative, so that H then turns out positive.

If $p_i = 0$, $p_i \log p_i = 0 \log 0$. Logarithm of 0 is minus infinity, but $0 \log 0$ is defined as 0 for convenience. If $p_i = 1$, $p_i \log p = 0$ again. Hence H is zero for $p = 0$ or 1, i.e. for constant characters, which is what one would expect. One can also show that H is a maximum for any m when all p_i are the same and equal to $1/m$. In other words, H is largest when all states are equally distributed. The maximum value is $\log m$. If $m = 2$, we can confine H to the range 0 to 1 by using logarithms to the base 2. For larger m, the range of H is 0 to $\log m$. If one wanted to confine H always to the range 0 to 1, then logarithms to base m can be used for characters with m states, because $\log_m m = 1$. This is in effect just the same as multiplying H by a normalising constant.

Index